Swiss Ball Applications for Orthopedic & Sports Medicine

A GUIDE FOR HOME EXERCISE PROGRAMS UTILIZING THE SWISS BALL

First Edition

by Joanne Posner-Mayer, PT

Published by

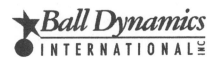

Ball Dynamics
INTERNATIONAL INC

Printed on recycled paper
in the United States of America .

Library of Congress Number 95-076115
ISBN Number 0-9645341-4-2

Design and Production by Sandra Caudill
Edited by Jauna Hyer and Joanne Posner-Mayer, PT
Illustrations:
Exercise illustrations by Marianna Amicarella
Optimal spine illustrations printed with
permission from Ritmobil srl, Ledraplastic, Inc.

Published by:
Ball Dynamics International, Inc.

1-800-752-2255

Dedication

This book is dedicated to my beloved family who enriched my childhood with fascinating stories about Europe which instilled me with the motivation and desire to explore it myself. I would like to honor the memory of my grandparents, Emma and Julius Krüger, who were victims of the Holocaust, my father, Jerry Posner who came to America as a young boy and my aunt and uncle, Anna Marie and Kurt Heimbach, who immigrated as young adults.

Also, I would like to express my deepest love and gratitude to my mother, Hanna Krüger-Ohr, my husband, Dale Mayer, and our son, Jason Alan. Without them, I would not have had the opportunity to focus my energy on this material collected and created during my first twenty years as a physical therapist.

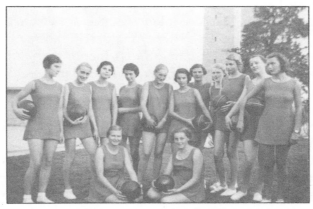

Hanna Krüger, 17 years old (bottom left) participating in the opening ceremony of the 1936 Olympics, Berlin, Germany. See Hanna on cover picture at 76 years old still using balls for exercise!

Acknowledgments

I would like to take this opportunity to thank Mr. Duane Saunders, PT, for encouraging me to publish this book and for supporting my videos. To Ledraplastic and the Cosani family, Grazie!, for your ongoing support and trust in my abilities.

Since this is my first book, I would like to thank all those who inspired me to become a physical therapist, contributed to my professional education and gave me instruction on ball techniques. This includes: Lillian Covillo and Friedan Parker, founders of the Colorado Ballet, Mrs. Eleanor Westcott, my enthusiastic Therapeutic Exercise instructor, Dr. Karl Kobsa, for my first PT position in Switzerland, Dr. Bruno Baviera, Director of the Physical Therapy School in Bad Schinznach, for his continued support and ideas, Karl and Berta Bobath and NDT instructors for introducing their therapeutic techniques and the ball to America and the therapists who pioneered ball techniques in Switzerland: Dr. Susanne Klein-Vogelbach, Maria Kucera and Mary Quinton for their knowledge . My thanks to Dennis McGimsey, owner of Integrated Medical, Inc. for the opportunity to present my ball class in five states. Also, I appreciate the opportunity given to me by The Jimmie Heuga Center to develop a therapeutic ball exercise class for their program for people with Multiple Sclerosis.

I would also like to thank these physical therapists for their teamwork on adapting my program to their specialities and for presenting with me at the various conferences and national conventions: Lee Day, Joan Gunther, Merry Lester, Patty McCord, Ginni Patterson, Mary Jean Taylor and Ray Vigil. Thank you Beate Carrière, PT, Paul Christensen, PT, Gay Girolami, PT, Kathie Hanson, PT, Marika Molnar, PT, Sandi Pomeroy, PT, and occupational therapists, Dr. Josephine Moore and Diane and Jeff Crabtree, for your knowledge, friendship and support. To my long-standing Swiss therapist friends, Maria DeMarmels, Karl Hodel, Susanne Niedermann, Theres Wagner, and German therapists Jutta Sternberg and Vera Waluga-Vielen Dank!

A special thanks to Janet Santopietro, Anne Spalding and Shirley Stafford, innovative early childhood educators, for inviting me to lecture with them to other teachers on ball uses for the school rooms as well as Physical Education classes. Thanks to Marianna Amicarella and Lindsay Zappala for their enthusiasm in applying the ball exercises to their treatment programs based on the Pilates approach and for presenting with me in the dance and fitness world. Also, thank you Lindsay for your collaboration on the FitBall® exercise video and manual. Marianna, thank you for your input and artistic ability.

Finally, I would like to gratefully acknowledge Jauna Hyer, for her invaluable assistance in preparing and editing this manuscript, and Sandra Caudill for her artistic contribution to the design and production of this book.

About the Author

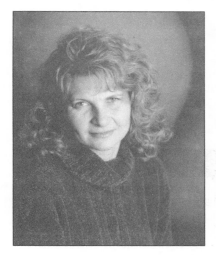

Joanne Posner-Mayer is a 1973 graduate of the University of Colorado Physical Therapy School. Due to lack of positions for therapists in Colorado at that time, she traveled to Switzerland on vacation and was successful in acquiring employment at the Stadtspital Triemli (City Hospital of Zürich). During her seven years of practicing in Switzerland, Joanne was able to learn from many therapists trained by Dr. Susanne Klein-Vogelbach and Frau Maria Kucera, PT. Besides working in the hospital and teaching at the in-house PT school with Frau Kucera, Joanne was able to attend manual therapy classes taught by Freddy Kaltenborn, D.O. She completed her Bobath (NDT) training in Bern, Switzerland under Mary Quinton, PT and Dr. Elsbeth Köng in 1978 and took a position at the Graubunden Foundation for Cerebral Palsy Children in Chur, Switzerland. This center was instrumental in implementing the first ski program for physically challenged children. This program has become a model for such programs throughout the international rehabilitation community.

In 1980, Joanne spent six months working at the University Orthopedic Hospital in Copenhagen, Denmark where she presented her first "Swiss Ball" class at a time when the ball was unknown there for orthopedic uses. Upon returning to the US, she worked in several different clinical settings from general hospital to home health and private practice while continuing her professional education in manual therapy. She instructed NDT techniques at the University of Colorado PT School from 1984-86 and often taught "Swiss Ball" inservices at facilities where she worked. In 1989, she became Director of Education at Integrated Medical, Inc. and began teaching "Swiss Ball" workshops on orthopedic techniques in her seminar "Therapeutic Exercises with the Gymnastic Ball".

Since 1989, she has presented hundreds of lectures and workshops on therapeutic applications using the "Swiss Ball". She has been a guest speaker at numerous PT, OT, ACSM and ATC state conventions. She has presented alone and in conjunction with colleagues at national conventions for the American Physical Therapy Association, Neuro-Developmental Treatment Association, National Association for the Education of the Young Child and American Alliance for Health, Physical Education, Recreation and Dance. In the past eight years, she has been a guest lecturer at the University of Colorado PT Program as well as at many PTA and COTA schools in Colorado. In addition, Joanne has lectured in Mexico, Canada, Brazil and Europe including presenting at the Brazilian Physiotherapy National Congress and the International Congress on Physical Activity, Aging and Sports in Germany.

In 1990, she founded Ball Dynamics International, Inc. to develop educational material on "Swiss Ball" use and to alleviate the shortage of "Swiss Balls" at that time by directly importing them. She has produced three videos on "Swiss Ball" use including: "Orthopedic, Sports Medicine and Fitness Applications Using the 'Swiss' Ball", "Spinal Stabilization Using the Swiss Ball" in conjunction with Merry Lester, PT, and "FitBall®-The Balanced Workout", a low-impact aerobics/conditioning video co-authored by Lindsay Ross. In 1993, Joanne translated Frau Kucera's Gymnastik mit dem Hüpfball (Exercises with the Gym-Ball) first published in 1974. In 1994, she and Lindsay Ross released the "FitBall® Exercise Manual". Joanne has recently released a computer program featuring this collection of ball exercises and is currently co-authoring the book "Kids on the Ball", a book designed for physical educators and teachers wanting to implement Swiss Ball use in schools.

FOR MORE INFORMATION ON SWISS BALL SEMINARS...

Contact: Joanne Posner-Mayer, PT

c/o   Ball Dynamics International, Inc.
            1-800-752-2255
or e-mail at **bdi@qadas.com**

OTHER PRODUCTS BY JOANNE POSNER-MAYER, PT...

Orthopedic, Sports Medicine and Fitness Applications Using The Swiss (Gymnic®) Ball video

This video demonstrates how to use ball exercises safely and effectively with clients of all ages and abilities. Segments include: joint and spinal mobility, static and dynamic strengthening, proprioception and kinesthetic training and cardiovascular fitness. 90 minutes.

Spinal Stabilization Utilizing the Swiss Ball video in collaboration with Merry Lester, PT

This video will educate you about instability and exercises using the Swiss ball which can add to your existing stabilization exercise program. The curriculum includes exercises starting with the patients acute/beginning phase and will progress to challenge healthy individuals or trained athlete. 35 minutes.

FitBall®-The Balanced Workout video in collaboration with Lindsay Ross, A.C.E. Certified

This 60 minute video is a fun and unique approach to low impact aerobics and total body fitness. While challenging your cardiovascular system, you will improve your balance, coordination and posture. The workout begins with an aerobic workout and finishes with stretching and strengthening. Also available, the **FitBall Workout Guide** has over fifty exercises for general fitness.

Therapeutic Ball Exercises- A Saunders' Exercises Xpress® Software

This software program provides a database of over 120 ball exercise illustrations and instructions divided into sections such as Spinal, Cardiovascular, Upper Extremity, Lower Extremity and Transfers. Using the PhysioTools sorting system, the user can employ a "pick and mix" approach to create individualized instruction sheet for each patient.

Exercises With The GymBall By: Maria Kucera, PT *Translated by: Joanne Posner-Mayer, PT*

An illustrated exercise manual of over 270 exercises including partner and group exercises. This is a good source for physical education teachers or therapists who are looking for high level activities.

Kids On The Ball book co-authored with physical education teachers-Anne Spalding, Linda Kelly and Janet Santopietro. The first instructional book for physical education teachers, early childhood educators and therapists who would like to integrate the balls into their school system for physical education and in the classroom setting.

Therapeutic Ball Exercises card deck-
Joanne Posner-Mayer's ball exercises in an easy to use format to photocopy for home programs.

Table of Contents

AMAZING!
Flat Abs In 3 Weeks

Every woman wants a tummy that's tight and toned. Now, in ten minutes and five moves, Jim Karas shows you how to get it.

Y ou've done floor crunches. You've bought infomercial gadgets. You've even cut back on calories. But still the midsection bulge remains. Is a widening waistline simply a fact of getting older? Absolutely not. But getting trim requires targeting the right muscles—and that's not always easy to do. Luckily, one piece of exercise equipment—a big, round ball—can put tummy troubles behind you for good.

Exercise balls offer a new approach to the ab-flab dilemma. While traditional crunches work only your stomach muscles—which gives you firmness but also shortens the muscle fibers (so your stomach looks firm but not flat)—ball exercises work your back muscles along with your abdominals. (Your torso is elevated by the ball, so moving in one direction activates ab muscles; moving in the other uses your lower back.) By working your back muscles, you're stretching or elongating your abs. The result: Using the ball, you'll look taller, leaner, and firmer much faster than you would if you did regular crunches.

This easy, five-exercise routine focuses on what fitness pros call your core—the ab and back area we've just been talking about. The program is perfectly safe, even for beginners, but if you have a history of back problems, it's good to check with your doctor first. Also, if you have trouble keeping your balance at any time during these exercises, you can always place the ball against a wall for support. Devote ten minutes a day, every day for three weeks, and I guarantee you'll see changes in the size and sleekness of your midsection. So go get your flat abs—and have a ball!

PHOTOGRAPHS BY MATTHEW RODGERS. Hair and makeup by Elisa Flowers at Bernstein and Andriulli. Styling by Kellan Whiteman. Sisal rug from Pottery Barn.

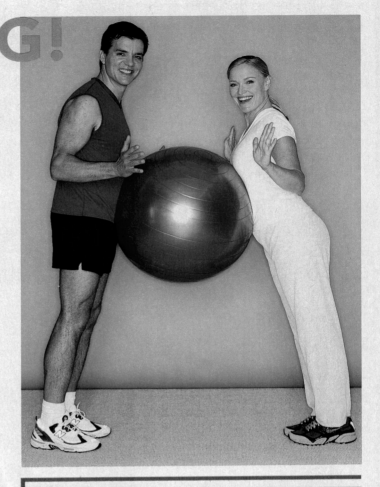

THE 10-MINUTE FLAT-AB PLAN

For each exercise, perform 12 to 15 repetitions.

1. BACK EXTENSION Lie facedown on top of the ball, legs extended behind you in a V, toes touching the floor. Place hands on either side of your head (1a). Slowly exhale and arch your body up (1b). Hold, then slowly inhale as you release. **TRAINING TIP:** Squeeze your shoulder blades as you lift.

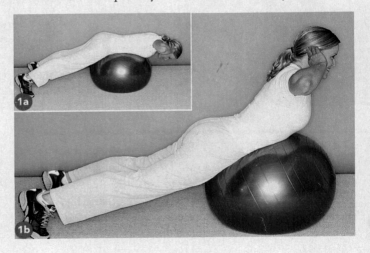

1a

1b

2. BALL BRIDGING Sit on the ball. Walk feet forward until your head, neck, and shoulders are supported on the ball. Keep your bottom just above the floor. Bend knees, keep feet shoulder-width apart, toes pointed forward (2a). Exhale and lift your hips so that they're in line with your knees (2b). Inhale; return to position 2a. **TRAINING TIP:** Squeeze your bottom and ab muscles as you lift.

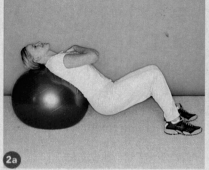
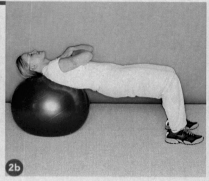

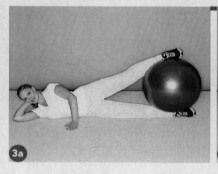
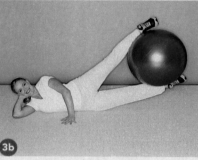

3. OBLIQUES TONER Lie on your side with the ball between your feet (3a). Resting your head on one hand, slowly lift both legs, squeezing the ball to keep it in place (3b). Exhale as you lift; inhale as you lower your legs to the starting position. Repeat on the other side. **TRAINING TIP:** Contract the sides of your waist (your obliques) as you lift.

4. DIAGONAL STRETCHES Lie facedown on top of the ball with your legs extended shoulder-width apart, toes on the floor (4a). Slowly lift and extend both your right arm and left leg, reaching out with your hand and pointing your toes (4b). Hold, then repeat on the other side. **TRAINING TIP:** If this exercise feels too strenuous, practice it first on the floor without using the ball.

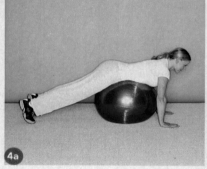
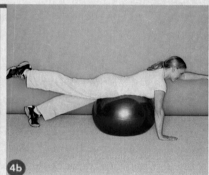

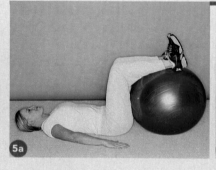
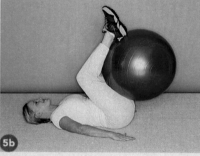

5. LOWER AB REVERSES Lie on your back, knees bent and feet on top of the ball (5a). Grip the ball between your heels and your bottom. Slowly exhale and raise hips off the floor, keeping tension on the ball as you bring it toward your chest (5b). Inhale and release. **TRAINING TIP:** Don't arch your lower back—keep it pressed to the floor.

GET A WORKOUT WHILE SITTING DOWN That's right: Because of the ball's rounded top and no rest for your back, simply sitting on it forces your abdominal muscles to work hard. Start out with five minutes of sitting (feet shoulder-width apart, toes forward, abs tight, and back straight) and build up to an hour. You can even do it while watching TV. Sound easy? Sit before you smirk.

For more fitness ideas, read The Business Plan for the Body *by Jim Karas (Three Rivers Press).*

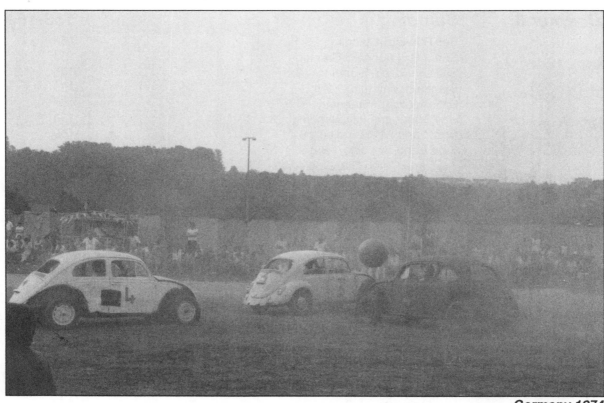

Germany 1974

History of the Swiss Ball

In the 2nd century A.D., Galen, an influential Greek philosopher and physician, wrote that exercising with a ball "can stir the enthusiast or the slacker, can exercise the lower portions of the body or the upper, some particular part rather than the whole, or it can exercise all the parts of the body equally...is able to give the most intense workout and the gentlest relaxation" (Sweet, 1987). Galen also points out "The best athletics of all are those which not only exercises the body but are able to please the spirit" (Sweet, 1987). Obviously, the benefits of exercising with balls have been recognized for centuries. The "Swiss Ball" is a unique, functional tool for therapists because people of all ages and cultural backgrounds associate balls with play and recreation. In clinical settings, the large ball has been found to increase client enjoyment and compliance with home exercise programs.

The "Swiss Ball", as it is known today, originated in 1963 when an Italian manufacturer, Mr. Aquilino Cosani, started producing toys made of vinyl instead of rubber. He developed techniques to make large yellow, orange and green (Gymnastik™) balls and sold them in Europe. In 1981, the company was divided and Mr. Cosani began producing a new line of balls and rolls with different standard colors such as red, blue and clear (Gymnic™). These two brands of therapy balls are widely used in hospitals and clinics around the world and balls manufactured by Mr. Cosani over twenty years ago are still in use.

Dr. Elsbeth Köng, a Swiss pediatrician who went to England to learn the Bobath method, was instrumental in setting the "Swiss Ball" in motion. In England, practitioners of the Bobath method did not usually treat children under two years of age. In Switzerland, Dr. Köng had the freedom and the insight to start treatment of newborns and infants. She invited Mary Quinton, an English physio-therapist, to work with her at the Inselspital in Bern, Switzerland in 1958. Together, Dr. Köng and Ms. Quinton developed programs using the Bobath method for early intervention which are now recognized internationally. Also, in 1966, Dr. Köng, along with Annemarie Ducommun, founded the first ski program for physically disabled children which continues to be practiced today. A book is now being published about this program and its methods.

Mary Quinton was the first qualified instructor of the Bobath method to practice in Switzerland. In the early 1960's, Ms. Quinton discovered the Gymnastik™ balls in Bern, Switzerland and began to integrate them into her treatments because she was able to facilitate better balance reactions and movement patterns compared to the large soft beach balls originally used in England. Ms. Quinton introduced the thick, vinyl balls to the Bobaths who also began using them and the balls gained the appellation "Bobath" balls. At 82 years old, Ms. Quinton continues to travel and teach pediatric Neuro-Developmental Treatment classes worldwide. At 73 years old, Dr. Köng is retired and often instructs with Ms. Quinton.

Dr. Susan Klein-Vogelbach was the founding director of the PT school in Basel, Switzerland from 1955 to 1974. She is known for developing the theory of movement called Functional Kinetics which is taught in all German speaking PT curriculums. She was introduced to the balls by a colleague who attended a Bobath class taught by Mary Quinton. Klein-Vogelbach was the first to use the balls with adults having orthopedic and other medical problems. She developed specific treatment techniques which she has incorporated into her Functional Kinetics classes since the mid 1960's. She first presented the ball exercises at the World Physical Therapy Congress in Amsterdam in 1970. Frau Klein-Vogelbach is now a doctor emeritus for her contributions to medical science. She has written numerous text books used in European PT schools and published "Ball Gymnastik for Functional Kinetics (Ballgymnastik zur funktionellen Bewegungslehre)" in 1980. It is presently being translated into English. However, a video of the exercises was released in English in 1993. At 84, she is still in private practice, teaching classes in Functional Kinetics and is presently writing a new book for therapists who treat musicians and another book on Gait Training.

In 1972, Maria Kucera, a Czech physical therapist and instructor for the two PT schools in Zürich, from 1970 to 1988, took a course from Klein-Vogelbach and was introduced to the ball. Kucera expanded a small repertoire of ball techniques to over 270 exercises in her book, Exercises with the Gym-Ball (Gymnastik mit dem Hüpfball). It has been available to European therapists since 1974 and and has recently become available throughout the US since its translation to English and Spanish in 1993. She is also the author of numerous other exercise textbooks used by PT schools throughout Europe. At the age of 73, Frau Kucera-Locher is now retired.

In the US, the large, vinyl balls were nicknamed "Swiss" because several US therapists saw the balls in clinics in Switzerland where the balls were first used for therapy and exercise by the before mentioned therapists. The "Swiss" ball was largely introduced to the US by the Bobaths themselves and two of their instructors, Joan Mohr and Pam Mullens, who also learned about ball use from Mary Quinton. They began bringing balls to the US to use in their own classes. In 1975, the first US company, Equipment Shop, began importing the balls.

For many years, the balls were used mainly in pediatric and neurological settings. However, as early as 1972, Beate Carrière, a German PT, and Kathie Hanson, an American PT who worked in Germany, were using the Functional Kinetics theory, teaching classes in the US and bringing balls over from Switzerland. Beate Carrière is the only practicing therapist in the US certified to teach Functional Kinetics by Dr. Klein-Vogelbach. Ms. Carrière teaches classes in the US, Germany and Iceland and practices in Los Angeles. In 1989, Joanne Posner-Mayer, PT, who practiced for seven years in Switzerland, began instructing US therapists on neurological, orthopedic and fitness applications of the "Swiss Ball" (See About The Author).

Many US therapists have been introduced to the use of "Swiss Ball" with spinal stabilization exercises. However, the ball was originally not a part of this program. Stemübungen, the original spinal stabilization method, was created in 1954 by Roswitha Brunkow, PT in Bad Homburg, Germany and eventually the techniques spread to Scandinavia. Some therapists who studied manual therapy techniques brought these exercise protocols back to the US. Also, in the late 1970's, many German speaking therapists started to attend the P.N.F. training program in Vallejo, California. These therapists shared some Swiss ball exercises with US physical therapists.

The ball's exact transition to the spinal stabilization method still has a nebulous origin starting in the San Francisco area. However, it can be traced back to Liz Schorn, a US physical therapist, learned the stabilization method working in West Germany at the Südeutsches Rehabilitationskrankenhaus. She was introduced to the ball when the clinic invited Frau Kucera to present a ball workshop. The clinicians combined portions of the two techniques and Ms. Schorn brought the resulting program to the San Francisco area when she returned in 1983. Due largely to her contact with numerous therapists and pioneering efforts in that area, the ball is now commonly associated with the spinal stabilization method in the US. "Swiss Balls" have been integrated into spinal stabilization classes taught by such therapists as: Paul Christensen, Dennis Morgan, Michael Moore, Greg Johnson and Vicki Saliba-Johnson, Mariano Rocabado and Beverly Biondi to mention a few.

Other therapists in the US have been creatively adapting "Swiss Balls" to their various settings. Elizabeth Noble has been using the balls in her post-partum program since 1982. Ilana Parker has created techniques using both foam rollers and "Swiss balls" based on her Feldenkrais background. She has been teaching classes in the US and Israel since 1988. Ninoska Gomez, Ph.D, a developmental psychologist and movement instructor in Canada and Latin America, is the creator of *Somatarhythms,* a program to refine somatic awareness using large, inflatable balls. Paul Callaway, PT, the first therapist to travel with the Professional Golf Association, has recently developed a successful program for golfers using "Swiss Balls" and elastic tubing to improve performance in their sport.

Since the late 1980's, the availability of education, both orthopedic and neurological, on therapeutic uses of the "Swiss Ball" has increased dramatically. Seminars, videos and books have become available from both US and European sources and balls are changing exercise protocols throughout the Western Hemisphere. Athletic trainers, coaches, personal trainers and physical education teachers have also begun to integrate the ball into their programs. Professional athletes such as football, baseball and basketball players, dancers, ice skaters and golfers are using the ball in their training programs. In 1991, the original fitness/wellness program, FitBall™, was created based on safe and effective therapy principles using the ball. Several other fitness programs have followed.

Since 1991, the ball has replaced chairs in schools for thousands of children in Europe due to increased education and information on the postural benefits of "active sitting" and back injury prevention. The classroom teachers found that: 1-hyper-active children became calmer and could focus for longer periods 2-other children could generally concentrate better. 3-hand writing skills improved for children with poor penmanship 4- children often showed a better understanding of subject material 5- disorganized children developed a better sense of organization (Illi, 1994). Studies are now in progress in the US testing the effectiveness of the ball for patients with Attention Deficit Disorder, balance disorders, hypotonicity, arthritis and osteoporosis. Numerous therapy clinics are now using the ball for rehabilitation of orthopedic, sports medicine, chronic pain and cardiac patients. Occupational rehabilitation facilities have begun to use the ball in conjunction with their traditional treatment methods. The possibilities for applying the "Swiss Ball" are growing as people in different fields discover its effectiveness.

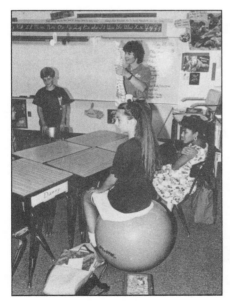

California Physical Therapist Marilyn Nishi, brings the Swiss balls to public schools to teach children the importance of good posture in a fun way. The children can experience the difference between passive sitting in a chair and active sitting on a ball.

**This history has been compiled by Joanne Posner-Mayer, PT, through her personal association with the above mentioned parties and personal research. She is continually updating this information and would appreciate receiving any correction or new information pertaining to the history of the "Swiss Ball".

A Motor Control Rationale for the Therapeutic Use of the Swiss Ball

by

Mary Jean Taylor, M.A., P.T., P.C.S.
Assistant Professor of Physical Therapy

Daemen College
Amherst, New York

Joan S. Gunther, Ph.D., P.T.
Associate Professor
Graduate Physical Therapy Program Director

Daemen College
Amherst, New York

Introduction

The Swiss Ball is a familiar and inexpensive piece of equipment found in many physical therapy clinics which can easily be incorporated into individual or group treatment sessions as well as home programs. The Swiss ball offers clinicians limitless options in evaluation and treatment of healthy as well as disabled individuals. Whether the patient has primary involvement in their musculoskeletal, neuromuscular or cardiopulmonary system, using the ball can add variety, challenge and fun to exercise programs. In healthy individuals, the ball may serve as a useful preventive tool, by promoting good health through exercise.

To guide therapists in the rational design of treatments or programs using the Swiss ball, it is helpful to work from a coherent theoretical foundation. Many physical therapists are advocating the use of information from the field of motor control as a framework from which to base our work. *Motor control* is the process by which the central nervous system uses "...current and previous information to coordinate effective and efficient functional movements..." [Horak, 1991] Reference to "previous information" underscores the importance of *motor learning* in generating movement. Motor learning is defined as "the process of acquiring the capability for producing skilled actions." [Schmidt, 1988]

The goal of this chapter is to integrate the practical applications of the Swiss ball into a contemporary theoretical framework based on a *systems model* of motor control and on principles of motor learning. It is not intended to be a comprehensive literature review, but rather a discussion of general principles.

Systems Model of Motor Control

According to the *systems model* of motor control humans can be viewed as multi-dimensional, complex, cooperative systems.[Scholz, 1990] From this perspective, motor behavior is an emergent property that results from the combined activity in all the functionally related subsystems. [Kamm, et. al., 1990] The efficiency of motor behavior depends upon the integrity of all the interacting subsystems. Functional movement, that is, movement aimed at performing a particular goal-directed task, emerges from the interaction between intrinsic systems:

- cognitive-limbic
- cardiopulmonary
- musculoskeletal
- neuromuscular
- sensoriperceptual

plus extrinsic physical characteristics of the environment and environmental forces; and the individual's morphology (see Figure 1.1). For example, the ability to ride a bicycle successfully depends upon the individual having sufficient interest and motivation to use this mode of transportation; endurance to ride a functional distance; strength in multiple muscle groups to overcome friction

Figure 1:1 Dynamic systems model of a biological organism. (Adapted from Horak, 1991. Reprinted with permission of the American Physical Therapy Association).

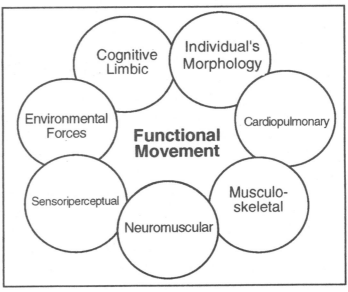

© 1995 by Joanne Posner-Mayer, PT

7

from the support surface or to negotiate changes in inclination of the support surface; muscle and joint flexibility to actively move through required ranges; and ability to recruit muscle synergies reciprocally as well as to disassociate right and left lower extremities. The individual must also have appropriate balance to maintain body stability on this dynamic device, which in turn depends on the integrity of visual, somatosensory, and vestibular systems as well as coordination of balance strategies. In addition, success and safety with bicycle riding will be dependent on the individual's perception of his body in space in relation to stationary and moving objects in the immediate environment. Finally, we need to consider whether the bicycle fits the individual appropriately. Performance will be altered if the bicycle is too small or too large. All of these factors operating simultaneously contribute to successful bicycle riding.

Systems theory incorporates the notion of order emerging from *"chaos"* in describing motor behavior. With chaos or randomness, there are many potential outcomes. Each subsystem which contributes to the final motor output (musculoskeletal, cardiopulmonary,...) has variability inherent within it. In the case of a healthy biological system, this variability results in great flexibility in potential movement strategies available to meet the demands within our environment. Biological systems are constantly challenged to reorganize, that is, to find order and stability. *Optimization* is the search for the best possible solution. With respect to movement, the optimal outcome will be the most efficient motor behavior that accomplishes the task. If potential choices are limited, the search is narrowed and a sub-optimal solution may result. This is often the case with our patients who have limited movement options for any of a wide variety of reasons. [Kamm, et. al., 1990]

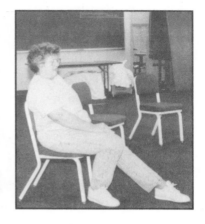

Note the sitting posture of the women with and without back support. Chaos is introduced when the women is asked to sit on the ball, a dynamic surface which is relatively unfamiliar. Of the many possible outcomes or choices, this individual chooses the optimal strategy. From a therapeutic stand point, the most erect posture is optimal. If the individual were to remain in her preferred posture, a posteriorly tilted plevis and thoracic kyphosis, more muscle activity would actually be required to maintain a sitting position on the ball.

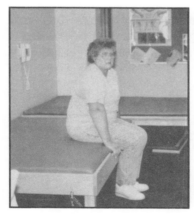
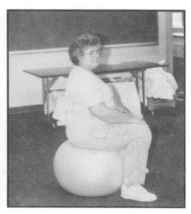

As therapists, we evaluate and identify impairments in one or more systems in our patients which result in less efficient or unsuccessful motor performance. From an evaluation standpoint, observing a patient while he or she is engaged in performing dynamic activities with the Swiss ball (eg. bouncing while sitting on the ball) can provide us with useful insights about complex interrelated factors governing movement, for example, symmetry, balance, muscle and joint flexibility, strength, and so on. Through treatment we attempt to optimize function of the compromised system(s) and thereby improve the movement outcomes. The ball, by virtue of its versatility, can be incorporated into our treatments to influence many of the biological subsystems that contribute to effective movement. The following chapters provide many safe and effective ball techniques that are available to improve muscle flexibility, joint range of motion, sensory-perceptual integrity, alertness, strength, endurance, coordination, and balance.

Information Processing and Memory

The systems approach to motor control reminds us that we should look at multiple systems or variables. However, we should remember that the central nervous system (CNS) serves as the common integrative element that ties them all together (Figure 1.2). The central nervous system does this by first defining the goal or task. For example, do I want to bring a glass of water to my mouth and take a drink? Next, CNS mediated perceptual processes evaluate the starting conditions under which the task is to be carried out. Among starting conditions we include both significant or *regulatory* stimuli [Gentile, 1987];as well as intrinsic stimuli related to the spatial orientation of the body, motivational factors, and the like. In our example, we might note that the glass is sitting on a table at a particular distance from us, that our dominant hand is holding a fork, and that we are thirsty. The context is also filled with irrelevant or ***non-regulatory*** stimuli which may confuse or distract the individual from completing the task efficiently. An example of such a non-regulatory stimulus

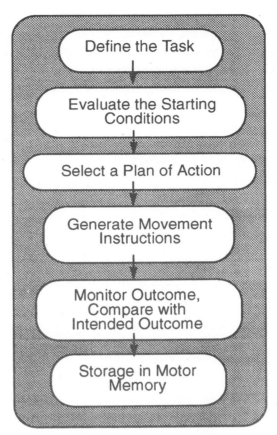

Figure 1:2 *Information Processing Model of Movement. The central and peripheral nervous system play a critical role at each stage of the process.*

might be a dog barking at the front door. Next, through CNS activity, we select a plan of action (response selection) and generate instructions for executing the movement that will lead to task completion. The more variable the conditions under which response selection occurs, the more potential choices there are for a successful movement strategy and the longer it takes to make the choice [Schmidt, 1988]. Movement generation occurs as the central and peripheral nervous systems activate muscles with the appropriate timing and with the proper kinetics. As the movement progresses, and/or after movement completion, the CNS monitors and compares actual movement outcome with the intended outcome. Did I successfully drink from the glass? Am I still thirsty? Finally, the degree of successfulness of the motor performance in achieving the goal and the motor program used in the behavior are consolidated and stored in memory.

Neurophysiological and behavioral studies have provided many insights into the role of the CNS in this information processing - movement generation - evaluation sequence. First, consider an individual's ability to identify the starting conditions in which a motor act is to be carried out. Stimulus identification requires accurate sensory reception and perceptual processing. Interestingly, the development of normal sensation appears to require *active* movement. Kittens, for example, who are moved passively in their environment fail to demonstrate normal visually guided motor behaviors (eg. parachute reaction and blinking to a rapidly approaching visual stimulus)[Held, 1965]. Active movement also appears to be critical for the ability of humans to adapt their motor output to persistently altered sensory input. Consider an individual attempting to descend a flight of stairs for the first time wearing bifocal glasses. The distorted visual perception of distance, so disturbing initially, disappears over a short time period due to the remarkable adaptability of visual perceptual processes which occur during movement. This anecdotal finding has been confirmed by experiments in which humans who wear prism lenses for a period of days can adapt their motor output to compensate for visual input which systematically distorts the direction or location of objects in space. [Rosenbaum, 1991]

Sensory deficits (eg. visual, somatosensory, auditory, etc.) are commonly encountered in clinical practice. We typically expect to see sensory changes in the neurologic patient. However, we should also remember that sensory impairments may accompany other conditions, for example, surgery, trauma and aging (see Figure 1.3). Normal sensory input (S) enters the central processor (CNS) and results in normal motor output (following line x to M). Altered sensory input (S') enters the central processor and results in abnormal motor output (following line y to M'). The aim of physical therapy treatment would be to provide practice opportunities in which our patients could make use of central processing adaptations in the hope that abnormal sensory input would result

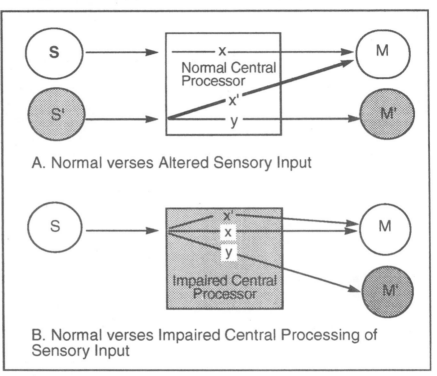

Figure 1:3 *Alterations in sensory input (A) or alterations in the central processing of information (B) result in altered motor output (M').*

A. Normal verses Altered Sensory Input

B. Normal verses Impaired Central Processing of Sensory Input

in normal or near normal motor output (following line x' to M). Based upon the experiments referred to above on sensory-motor adaptation, we might infer that active movement and the sensory feedback it generates are important in training our patients to adapt their motor output to compensate for altered sensory input.

With CNS damage, the normal flow of information processing (follow line x from S to M) has been disrupted to a greater or lesser degree. Altered central processing of sensory input (impaired central processor) results in abnormal motor output (following line y to M') despite the presence of normal peripheral sensory receptors (S). The goal of therapy is to provide practice opportunities that challenge the remaining information processing capabilities in the hope of bringing about as nearly normal motor output as possible (along line x' to M).

In the presence of altered sensory input or damaged central processing of sensory input, the Swiss ball provides the opportunity for a variety of active movements in conjunction with a great deal of movement-generated intrinsic sensory feedback. Theoretically, this should promote sensorimotor coordination. Response selection can be challenged by activities that involve throwing or weight bearing and balancing on a ball in a variety of active postures and tasks (refer to 6:14) because the individual interacting with the ball must quickly make correct choices to be successful. Variability between trials (the ball never does exactly the same thing twice) promotes flexibility in motor strategies because there are many successful ways to interact with the ball to accomplish a particular goal.

The CNS also provides for the storage of memories related to motor learning. Two types of memory have been described [Kandel and Schwartz, 1985]. *Declarative memory* is cognitive in nature, requires conscious attention, and is thought to be important in the early stages of motor learning. *Reflexive memory* has a more unconscious automatic quality and underlies balance and other well-learned motor behaviors.

Both declarative and reflexive memory can be called into play by training with the ball. For example, anyone sitting on the ball for the first time is challenged in a very cognitive way to maintain their upright sitting posture on the ball. At the same time, any available automatic movement strategies (righting and equilibrium reactions) are retrieved from reflexive memory. As training continues, the relative contribution of declarative memory diminishes and responses become more automatic. If, however, the task is altered to make it more difficult, for example by decreasing the base of support on the ball or increasing the speed of the activity, the need for cognitive processing again becomes necessary. The requirement of active attention to task performance makes the Swiss ball a useful therapeutic medium in cases where increasing a patient's cognition is itself an important goal of therapy.

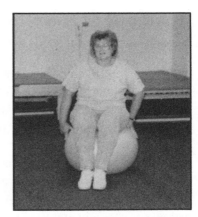

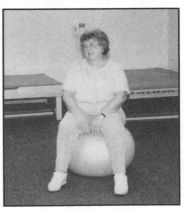

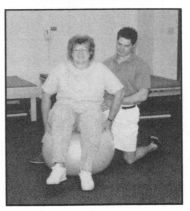

Both declarative and reflexive memory can be called into play by training on the ball. Initally, this woman is challenged in a very cognitive way to maintain her upright sitting posture on the ball. Simultaneously, any available automatic movement strategies are retrieved from reflexive memory. After serveral practice sessions, the contribution of declarative memory diminshes. If given a new motor challenge, in this case narrowing the base of support by altering lower extremity position, the need for cognitive processing again becomes necessary.

Task Analysis

As clinicians we attempt to achieve comprehensive movement rehabilitation of our patients. Therefore, we must ask ourselves critically, do we do a thorough job? Gentile has proposed a classification of tasks which we can use as a theoretical framework for answering this question. Her classification is based upon the function the task needs to fulfill and the environmental context in which the task needs to be carried out [Gentile, 1987]. If we consider the functions of a task, they can be divided into those that result in *body stability* or *body transport*. With body stability the individual remains stable within his environment; whereas, with body transport, the individual is moving in his environment. Each of these categories can potentially occur in the presence or absence of manipulation (ie. skilled use of upper or lower extremities).

Based on environmental context, we can distinguish between open, intermediate and closed tasks. The simplest tasks are *closed tasks*. These are tasks in which regulatory stimuli are stable and predictable and there is no variability between trials. An example of a closed task would be transitioning from sit to stand from a dining room chair. The most complex tasks are *open tasks*. These are tasks in which the regulatory stimuli are moving and vary from trial to trial. Moving to catch a ball which is thrown randomly is an example of an open task. Intermediate tasks are those for which the regulatory stimuli are not moving but vary from trial to trial. There are many options for providing variability between trials, for example, you might vary the support surface or the size and weight of what you are manipulating. Transitioning from sit to stand from a variety of different types of chairs is an example of an intermediate task.

In summary, for closed tasks, motor behaviors leading to task completion are very similar from trial to trial. For intermediate and open tasks, greater diversity in motor strategies is needed to insure successful task completion over trials.

Table 1:1 Therapeutic activities using the Swiss ball in relation to Gentile's Taxonomy of tasks (Gentile, 1972).

MOVEMENT FUNCTION

ENVIRONMENTAL CONTEXT		BODY STABILITY	BODY STABILITY PLUS MANIPULATION	BODY TRANSPORT	BODY TRANSPORT PLUS MANIPULATION
	CLOSED	Sit on a mat	Sit on a mat and reach with the ball in your hands towards a stationary target	Sit <-->Stand from a mat	Sit <-->Stand holding onto a ball
	INTERMEDIATE: STATIONARY ENVIRONMENT WITH INTERTRIAL VARIABILITY	Sit on a mat versus on a chair versus on a bench	Sit on a mat and reach for different size balls	Sit <-->Stand from a variety of chairs	Sit <-->Stand from various chairs holding onto different sized balls each trial
	OPEN	Sitting on a ball	Sitting on a ball doing a PRE program with UEs	Sit <-->Stand from a ball	Sit <-->Stand from a ball to catch a thrown object

Gentile's theoretical framework is useful in reminding us of categories of movement and environmental contexts that often escape our attention in designing our treatments. Within the taxonomy, the complexity of tasks increases from the least complex (closed tasks, body stability, without manipulation) to the most complex (open tasks, body transport with manipulation). For our patients, the ability to cope in stationary invariant environments is necessary but not sufficient if we consider the high degree of variability present in real life situations. A clinic therapist who only provides exercise training lying on a mat or ambulation training within the physical therapy gym will not adequately prepare the patient to cope with the information processing demands placed upon the same patient when ambulating along a busy street.

The ball allows us to rehabilitate all categories of movement within Gentile's classification. Using the ball makes available a variety of practice conditions that vary in difficulty, from skills that emphasize body stability with manipulation in stationary environmental conditions (see closed tasks, Table 1.1) to skills involving body mobility and manipulation in environmental conditions where regulatory stimuli are moving and change from trial to trial (see open tasks, Table 1.1). Any task performed in weight bearing on the ball is characterized by variability from moment to moment because the ball is an unstable base of support and never reacts exactly the same way twice. Different size, firmness, and weights of balls enhance variability between trials. Upper extremity range of motion and strengthening activities may be made more functional if they incorporate manipulation and placing activities with balls. Information processing, particularly response selection and rapid reaction time essential to success in open tasks, is challenged when the patient must trap a moving ball or glide from side-to-side across a ball (see 8:12).

Motor Learning

Motor learning or relearning is key to establishing or restoring optimal movement patterns. The development of dysfunction and pathology from movement imbalance is a well-accepted principle in neurological rehabilitation. Even in individuals without significant neurological impairment, the production of faulty movement patterns has been suggested to contribute to the development of dysfunction and pathology. Instruction in proper movement patterns has been suggested as a key element in promoting biomechanically sound and efficient movements [Sahrmann, S. 1987].

Motor skill acquisition is thought to occur in stages [Fitts,1964; Gentile, 1972]. In general, the early stages are thought to be highly cognitive, require conscious attention, and verbal cues are often used to direct or prompt performance. Feedback is important in the early stages to evaluate the success of the motor strategy used in relation to the expected and actual task outcome. As practice continues, the learned behavior becomes more automatic in nature, requiring less conscious monitoring, less direction of our attention, and less examination of feedback. There is an increase in the ease and efficiency with which the movements are executed. As the learned skill becomes more automatic, it may be possible for the learner to engage in other behaviors simultaneously without experiencing a deterioration in the former behavior. Gentile has used the terms *"fixation"* in referring to learning which narrows the range of performance outcomes resulting in increased consistency of performance (eg. signing one's name); and *"diversification"* to describe the acquisition of a more flexible motor strategy that is quickly adaptable to changing regulatory environmental conditions (eg. sitting on a ball and drawing the letters of the alphabet with your foot. See chapter 6:14).

Whether fixation or diversification should be the goal of treatment depends upon the particular task in question and the conditions under which the patient will have to carry it out in his/her own environment. The occurrence of fixation and diversification as a result of training depends upon the conditions under which training takes place. In retraining lost or impaired movements, it is important for the patient to practice the movements under conditions that mimic those in which the movements will ultimately need to be carried out. [Schmidt, 1991] Bernstein's work emphasizes the profound effects upon movement exerted by contextual factors like inertia, momentum and gravity.[Turvey, et. al., 1982] Swiss ball treatment activities can be used to challenge our patients to work towards either fixation or diversification, as appropriate, and to manage environmental variables. Practicing closed tasks utilizing the ball could be used to work on fixation. Practicing intermediate and open tasks with the ball facilitates the development of diversification. Bouncing on the ball at different intensities allows an individual to safely experiment with momentum and controlling his body against gravity, seeking strategies to manage both under the supervision of a therapist or trainer. Different degrees of inertia must be managed in order to trap a rolling ball in comparison to kicking a stationary ball and setting it in motion.

According to Bernstein, the acquisition of motor skill involves the development of *"coordinative structures"*--the functional linking together of different body segments.[Tuller, et. al., 1982] Coordinative structures are developed through practice and contribute to the automaticity of well-learned motor behaviors. Ball activities promote the development of coordinative structures since body parts are not being trained in isolation from one another as often occurs in traditional therapeutic exercise programs on a mat. When standing trapping a ball with the foot, axial postural muscles are activated simultaneously with extremity muscles to maintain the center of gravity over the base of support (see 6:15). This motor activity closely approximates the adaptive balance strategy used in avoiding a fall.

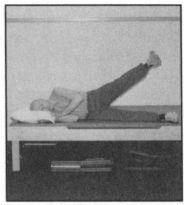

Feedback about the effectiveness of a movement is essential for motor learning. Generally, two kinds of feedback, intrinsic and extrinsic, have been identified. **Intrinsic feedback** is generated from one's position or movement and reported on by one's own senses, eg. somatosensory, vestibular, visual and auditory. **Extrinsic feedback** comes from sources outside the individual, for example, verbal cues about performance from a therapist or coach.[Schmidt, 1988] We learn efficient motor strategies from making motor errors. Ideally, errors are identified by relating intrinsic feedback from our performance to task accomplishment. This is based on the assumption that the sensory pathways that provide this information are intact. Under these conditions, caution must be taken to monitor the amount of extrinsic feedback we provide, as individuals may become dependent upon extrinsic cues and fail to be successful with movement behavior when they are absent.

Ball activities are useful in generating intrinsic feedback to the central nervous system. For example, sitting on and balancing

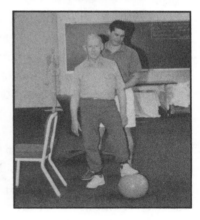

One may determine that the reason an individual is unstable in standing is in part due to hip abductor weakness. The individual may strengthen in the sidelying position; however based on the literature supporting development of coodinative structures and specificity of training, it may be more appropriate to work on strengthening in a unilateral stance position under dynamic environmental conditions.

on the ball provides vestibular input, somatosensory stimulation of pressure and joint receptors, visual stimulation and so on. The ball challenges an individual to utilize his intrinsic feedback which motor learning theorists have suggested is critical to motor learning.[Schmidt, 1988] We can take advantage of the dynamic properties of the ball to reduce verbal/manual cues (extrinsic feedback) about movement quality and elicit movement more automatically. For instance, for many clients who have trouble learning a posterior pelvic tilt based on instructions like "tuck your tummy and press your back into the table" can automatically accomplish the task when seated on a ball if they (or the therapist) roll the ball forward a small amount. In order to stay on the ball, the patient elicits a balance reaction, in this case, a posterior pelvic tilt. They now have an idea of the movement based on a motor memory generated from their intrinsic feedback. With continued practice opportunities, they may be able to elicit this movement with ease.

Treatment Applications

Range of Motion:

The integrity of a coordinative structure or an efficient movement sequence is dependent upon the available joint range and muscle flexibility. The ball may be used as an alternative or adjunct method to more traditional stretching techniques. In many cases, the ball provides a firm but comfortable weight bearing surface which supports the patient while stretching. Because of the dynamic qualities of the ball, the patient can move slowly in and out of their terminal range actively grading the degree of stretch and using gravity for assistance. A comprehensive guide of ranging activities with the ball is described and illustrated in Chapters 2, 5 and 6.

Increasing Strength:

Increasing muscle strength is an important factor in restoration of efficient movement behaviors. The ball may serve as an important piece of equipment in strengthening a wide variety of muscle groups in almost all exercise modes. For example, the ball can be used for isometric or isotonic exercises. The ball can be used as a weight for concentric or eccentric resistive exercise (see 8:7). In addition, the ball can be used as a fulcrum in weight bearing positions to lift the weight of body parts against gravity (see 3:3). In conjunction with work hardening activities, it can be used to optimize strength within a functional pattern. Closed kinematic chain activities can be trained in partial weight bearing positions by sitting or lying on the ball. With respect to specificity of training, the exercise routines utilizing the ball can be used to selectively rehabilitate phasic or tonic muscle fibers. The ball provides this phasic challenge in numerous ways including: lifting, catching, lying prone over the ball and walking out on your hands (see 5:5); as well as, protective and equilibrium reactions elicited in response to one's own movements on the ball. Tonic responses can be elicited in core (trunk) muscles in weight bearing activities simply by sitting on the ball, or in more advanced tasks like prone push-ups over the ball (see 5:2 & 5:3).

Most importantly, from a motor control perspective, strengthening is accompanied by retraining of the coordinative structure. Not only is the strength of individual elements increased, but each muscle is strengthened as part of a larger functional unit which involves development of optimal timing and the appropriate amount of force produced in contracting muscles.

Cardiovascular Training:

For many patients, one focus of treatment is to enhance or restore cardiopulmonary integrity. The ball can be incorporated into a sequence of aerobic therapeutic activities of increasing vigor. The patient might begin by simply sitting or bouncing on the ball and progressing to energetic, rhythmic routines incorporating upper and lower extremity movements. For a full description of cardiovascular and fitness exercises, see Chapter 1.

Sensory Perceptual Retraining:

The evaluation of sensory input is integral to motor performance and represents the way in which the individual identifies the regulatory stimuli in a particular situation. In addition, it is essential for providing feedback about the success of a motor strategy. A wide array of sensory input bombards the individual exercising with the ball.

Weight bearing on the ball is accompanied by somatosensory information generated by contact between the ball and weight bearing body segments. Activation of joint receptors and muscle spindles has been shown to occur due to the kinds of activities simulated by bouncing and transitioning on a ball.[Gaudin and Jones, 1989]

Widespread excitatory and inhibitory physiological effects can be obtained through vestibular stimulation by using the ball. The facilatory effects include increased tone in postural extensors as well as the elicitation of righting and equilibrium responses. The increased tone in back extensors and abdominals probably accounts at least in part for the improved alignment often noted in response to seated bouncing on the ball. Connections between vestibular nuclei and the reticular formation are thought to mediate increased general arousal and alertness. This may account for behavioral state changes of lethargic individuals during seated ball activities. Inhibitory vestibular influences on arousal or muscle tone can also be obtained on the Swiss ball by slowing the movement velocity or altering the position of the patient.[Umphred, 1990]

The dynamic nature of the ball leads to movement of the patient's body within space which is perceived by the visual, vestibular and somatosensory systems. The ability to stimulate these systems simultaneously allows you the opportunity to work on integration of multimodal sensory information which may be impaired in a wide range of conditions from learning disabilities [Montogomery, 1986] to chronic dizziness.[Telian, S. and Shepard, N., 1990] In the orthopedic . patient, use of the ball can be an effective treatment modality for providing proprioceptive information which is useful in movement re-education following injury or trauma.[Richardson and Iglarsh, 1994]

Balance:

Balance is not a unitary motor skill and there is presently no universally accepted definition or measurement of balance.[Berg, K., et al., 1989] Yet, therapists can certainly agree that the balance requirements vary depending upon the nature of the task and depending upon the environmental context in which the task is to be performed. For example, the balance requirements are quite different for sitting on a moving bus compared to sitting on a desk chair. Using Gentile's task analysis, we might say that balance performance depends upon whether the task environment is more open or closed. Indeed, a major factor in the increasing difficulty of tasks within the taxonomy is the extent to which rapid postural reactions need to be made automatically utilizing intrinsic sensory feedback. Use of the ball in addressing balance may be beneficial because it generates a great deal of intrinsic feedback and challenges the patient in a very unconscious way to make rapid postural adjustments thereby reinforcing the coordinative linkage between postural muscles.

Maintaining a high level of skill in balance activities requires constant challenge and practice. Inactivity results in loss of motor skill in balance which can in turn cause a fall. An individual aware that his balance is compromised becomes more fearful and avoids activities where his balance is challenged. The result is a cycle in which the fear leads to further inactivity (Figure 1.5). Alterations in any of the subsystems described previously in the systems model of motor control may lead to inactivity. Theoretically, maintaining a high level of activity should ensure the persistence of functional balance skills. Interventions using the ball can provide varying degrees of challenge to balance skills and progressively break the cycle of fear and inactivity at any age.

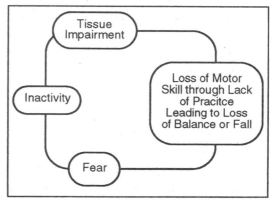

Figure 1.5 *The proposed relationship of inactivity to loss of balance.*

Postural Relearning:

Most therapists would agree that for effective postural relearning the individual must be actively engaged in an exercise routine which restores flexibility as well as muscle balance around the involved joint segments. Further, if we are to strengthen postural coordinative linkages, we need to consider if demands on the muscles are more phasic or tonic in nature. It has been suggested that postural demands require recruitment of tonic muscle fibers for sustained periods of time. [Oliver, J. Middleditch, A. 1991] It would then appear important to consider current exercise protocols and how effectively they challenge these core muscle groups. For example, if we consider the ability to maintain more neutral spinal alignment in sitting, emphasis should be placed on increasing strength and endurance in the multifidi and obliques rather than the phasic torque producing qualities of the erector spinae and rectus abdominus.

It is interesting to contemplate how much time our patients spend in supported sitting at school, in the office and at home. This may contribute to lack of spinal muscular endurance, development of muscular dysfunction and subsequent injury. In contrast to a chair which passively supports an individual's trunk, the ball represents a dynamic sitting surface which is ideal for enhancing postural muscle endurance.

Clinicians have noticed that in the absence of structural restriction sitting and/or bouncing on a ball appears to facilitate neutral spinal alignment. While it is clearly the case that one can still see postural deviations in individuals seated on a ball, the degree of postural deviation is often less than during supported sitting in a chair with arms and a back (or in standing unsupported.) Anecdotal observations suggest that if an individual sitting on a ball moves out of neutral alignment into a slouched position (posterior pelvic tilt), increased recruitment activity in abdominal and hip flexor muscles is required to sustain this position. An increase in muscle activity may also occur if an individual attempts to sustain a seated position on the ball with an excessive degree of lumbar lordosis. It would seem the most efficient position, requiring the least amount of muscle activity, is probably a neutral position midway between the two extremes. Typically, an individual finds this acceptable neutral range (optimization) as a result of sitting and bouncing on the ball without excessive guidance from the therapist providing they have the range and balance to maintain this position on the ball. From the perspective of a systems model of motor control, the body seeks the most efficient motor strategy it is capable of organizing.

Prevention and Fitness:

Quality of life is dependent upon maintained health of the mind and body. Participation in fitness programs influences the integrity of multiple body systems enhancing continued functional independence at home and within the community.[McArdle, et al., 1991] This is an important consideration particularly for the elderly population. Increasing emphasis is being placed on restorative and preventative health care programs for the elderly in an attempt to ensure higher quality of life and minimize costs within the health care system.[Vallbona, C. and Baker, S., 1984]

Ball activities can be incorporated into group or individual sessions for a wide range of individuals to influence performance of their cardiovascular, neuromuscular, and musculoskeletal systems. The ball adds novelty to pre-existing fitness programs keeping individuals interested and compliant with their exercises. In addition, even the most finely tuned individual can be challenged by the ball because of its dynamic qualities. The stronger and more balanced an individual, the more challenged they become as they narrow their base of support, increase their speed, their degree of weight shift, or height of their center of gravity on the ball. Exercise routines with the ball can be as gentle or as strenuous as the therapist or fitness instructor deems appropriate. Utilizing the full potential of the ball is a rewarding and exciting challenge to the creativity and ingenuity of the therapist, fitness instructor or client/patient.

Summary

The Swiss ball is a versatile treatment modality whose effectiveness can be viewed from a motor control and motor learning perspective. The Systems Model is one approach to motor control. Observing the way an individual interacts with the Swiss ball provides important evaluative information about the integrity of multiple systems. From a treatment perspective, the ball may be utilized to challenge particular systems where deficits are found. Movement occurs in the context of information processing, that is, evaluation of environmental stimuli, response selection and movement generation. Treatment with the Swiss ball challenges the efficiency and the flexibility of information processing capabilities. Task analysis is a way of conceptualizing the range of motor behaviors from very simple to highly complex activities requiring greater degrees of information processing. In training individuals to function as efficiently and independently as possible, we need to challenge them with motor behaviors representative of the full spectrum of tasks. Working with the Swiss ball provides opportunities to train movements throughout the entire classification of tasks. A key concept in motor learning is the development of "coordinative structures", that is, the linkage of body parts functioning together as an integrated unit. Use of the Swiss ball encourages the development of coordinative structures by requiring the simultaneous participation of multiple body areas as an individual works to balance on the ball. From a theoretical perspective, a sound rationale exists for use of the Swiss ball.

Glossary

body stability: the individual remains stable within his environment.

body transport: the individual is moving within his environment.

closed kinematic chain: when the distal segment of an extremity is fixed in a weight bearing position.

closed tasks: tasks in which the regulatory stimuli are stable and predictable; there is no variability between trials.

coordinative structures: muscle synergies which result in integrated control of muscles across multiple joints or body segments.

declarative memory: memory which involves conscious reflection for learning and recall.

diversification: learning which leads to flexible movement strategies and is essential to successful performance in open tasks.

fixation: learning which leads to a consistent movement strategy and is primarily associated with successful performance in closed tasks.

Motor control: refers to production of efficient motor behaviors for successful task completion.

Motor learning: the process of acquiring flexible strategies which allow an individual to consistently achieve a motor goal.

non-regulatory stimuli: extraneous sensory information which needs to be ignored when establishing a motor strategy.

open tasks: tasks in which the regulatory stimuli are moving and vary from trial to trial.

optimization: arriving at the best motor solution to accomplish a motor task.

regulatory stimuli: pertinent sensory information important for establishing a motor strategy.

reflexive memory: memory which has an automatic quality and does not depend on conscious reflection for learning or recall.

systems model of motor control: the interaction of multiple subsystems within the body to produce movement.

taxonomy: Classification or arrangement of .

Motor Control Rationale Bibliography

Berg, K., et al., 1989 Measuring balance in the elderly: preliminary development of an instrument. Physiother. Canada, 41. 304-311.

Fisher, N.M. et al., 1991 Muscle rehabilitation in impaired elderly nursing home residents. Arch Phys Med & Rehab, 72: 181.

Gaudin and Jones, 1989 Human Anatomy and Physiology. San Diego: Harcourt Brace Jovanovich.

Gentile, 1987

Gentile, 1987 Movement Science. Foundations for Physical Therapy in Rehabilitation. Carr, J. and Shepher, R. Eds. Aspen Publ.: Rockville, Md. held, 1965 Plasticity in sensory-motor systems. Sci. Amer., 213(5): 84-94.

Kamm, et al., 1990

Kamm, et al., 1990 A dynamical systems approach to motor development. Phys Ther.,70:763-775.

Kandel and Schwartz, 1985 Principles of Neural Science. Elseview: New York.

McArdle, et al., 1991 Exercise Physiology. Energy, Nutrition, and Human Performance. Philadelphia: Lea & Febiger. (Third edition)

Montgomery, 1986 Sensorimotor Integration for Developmentally Disabled Children: A Handbook. WPS: Los Angeles.

Richardson and Iglarsh, 1994 Clinical Orthopaedic Physical Therapy. Philadelphia, Saunders.

Rosenbaum, 1991 Human Motor Control. Academic Press, Inc.: San Diego.

Sahrmann, S., 1987 Posture and muscle imbalance: faulty lumbar-pelvic alignment and associated musculoskeletal pain syndromes. Postgraduate Advances in Physical Therapy.

Schmidt, 1988 Motor Control and Learning. A Behavioral Emphasis. Champaign, Ill. Human Kinetics Publ. Inc.

Schmidt, 1991 Motor Learning Principles for Physical Therapy. In Contemporary Management of Motor Control Problems. Proceedings of the II Step Conference. Foundation for Physical Therapy: Fredericksburg.

Scholz, 1990 Dynamic Pattern Theory: some implications for therapeutics. Phys ther.,70: 827-843.

Telian, S. and Shepard, N., 1990 Habituation therapy for chronic vestibular dysfunction. Otolaryngology Head and Neck Surgery, 103(1),

Tuller, et al., 1982 The Bernstein perspective: II. The concept of muscle linkage or coordinative structures. In J.A.S. Kelso (Ed.), Human motor behavior: An introduction. Hillsdale, N.J.: Erlbaum.

Turvey, et al., 1982 The Bernstein perspective: II, The concept of muscle linkages or coordinative structures. In J.A.S. Kelso (Ed.), Human motor behavior: An introduction. Hillsdale, N.J.: Erlbaum.

Umphred, 1990 Neurological Rehabilitation. St. Louis: Mosby.

Motor Control Rationale Index

This book is primarily a tool for therapists to design home programs for patients using ball exercises prescribed and practiced during supervised therapy sessions.** It also includes informative chapters to instruct therapists on the other aspects of ball use. However, any healthy individual can use this manual to learn and perform the exercises themselves for fun, fitness and injury prevention. The exercise instructions are designed for the general public to understand, where necessary, more technical terms are used (See Glossary, page 198-199). Be sure patients understand all terms used on their exercise sheets.

The chapter titles indicate the overall goal of the exercises in that chapter. However, any exercise in which the ball supports the body contains a balance component. Several exercises, although grouped in a specific chapter, can be used for other goals. For instance, Squat and Arch, in chapter 2, is a supported spinal extension stretch but can also be used for strengthening and proprioception of the hips, knees and ankles. Therapists are encouraged to look for a variety of applications for each exercise.

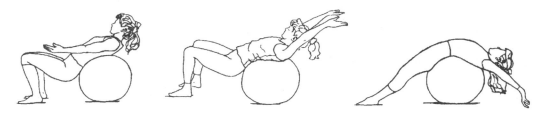

The exercises have been written with instructions and drawings to clarify *starting positions* and *movements* along with suggested *modifications* and *progressions*. Each chapter is arranged beginning with the most gentle exercises and progressing to the most difficult. Therapists need to use their clinical expertise to decide the number of exercises given to each patient as well as the level of the exercise which the patient is capable of performing safely. The number of repetitions, weights and frequency along with duration for stretches have been left for the clinician to prescribe.

Every patient needs a customized program for their injury/condition.

Patients usually comply better when they understand the goal of an exercise. The clinician has a "Purpose/Goal" field to fill in for each patient. Many of the exercises are beneficial for numerous conditions (strengthening, balance, stretching) and body parts (back, hip, knee). Therefore, it is important for the therapist to clarify the individual's goal.

SAMPLE:

Hold____Seconds / Weights____ / Repeat____Times / Do____Times/day

Purpose/Goal:_____

When Prescribing a Swiss Ball Home Program:

It is strongly recommended for the therapist to review safety instructions with the patient.

Each patient should be given the following pages:
1.   Suggested Sitting (Optimal) Posture (page 27/28).
2.   Suggested Inflation Instructions (See Appendix, page 193).
3.   Cleaning and General Safety Instructions (See Appendix, page 194).
4.   When applicable, give the instructions for commonly used pumps (See Appendix, page 195).

The ball is one of the most enjoyable, affordable and versatile exercise tools available. It has been used with low level neurological patients and acute pain patients as well as with healthy school children and world class athletes. These exercises can also be applied to people of all ages from toddlers to seniors and adapted for use with groups of differing abilities. There are very few contraindications or precautions for using the ball.

Contraindications

1.   Patient fear. This is rare but can usually be overcome with demonstration and assurances from the therapist.
2.   Complaints of increased pain, dizziness and/or impairment symptoms.
3.   Disease or injury-specific exercise contraindications

Precautions

1.   Guard patient adequately.
2.   Patient will fatigue quicker as balance is constantly challenged.
3.   Do not fatigue patient because they are enjoying exercises.
4.   Monitor signs of cardiac distress.
5.   Vertebral mobility exercises may flare up symptoms of Degenerative Joint Disease.

Benefits: In clinical use, the ball has been found to increase all of the following:

•   Mobility
•   Stability
•   Balance
•   Strength
•   Circulation
•   Coordination
•   Postural Control
•   Cardiovascular Fitness
•   Vital Capacity of Lungs
•   Nutrition to Body Structures
•   Enjoyment and Compliance with Exercise Program

The ball is unique from other forms of exercise because it:

- activates the whole body to maintain balance.
- facilitates midline orientation.
- distributes body weight over a relatively large yet dynamic base of support.
- creates two bases of support for the patient, the mobile ball over the stable floor.
- lowers the height of the body allowing equilibrium reactions and difficult movement patterns to be elicited at a relatively safe distance from the floor.
- forces the body to work at the level of its weakest part because substitutions and/or compensations with a stronger part pushes alignment off center.
- integrates body strengthening, mobilization and coordination as they exist in functional activities.

Difficulty of the exercises can be increased by making one or several of the following changes.

1. Decrease base of support
2. Increase lever arm
3. Increase distance traveled
4. Increase speed of movement
5. Add resistance- resistive band, free weights or manual resistance
   Conversely, difficulty can be reduced by making the opposite changes.

When a patient is given a home program using the ball, inform them that even just sitting on the ball is an exercise. Encourage them to use the ball as a chair as often as possible to promote "active (unsupported) sitting". People will generally not just sit on the ball but will start rocking, bouncing and stretching because it feels good. If they start bouncing for extended periods of time in optimal posture, they can improve the endurance of the postural muscles. Vigorous bouncing combined with arm and leg movements will increase heart rate and can improve cardiovascular fitness when performed at the proper level for an adequate amount of time. If patients are unable to set aside time during a busy day to perform their exercise program, suggest sitting on the ball while talking on the phone or watching television. **Keep in mind that unsupported sitting is an endurance activity. Therefore, start slowly and increase the duration of activity as able.** (If the patient performs an exercise during each television commercial, they will have easily completed many exercises).

There are numerous elementary schools throughout Europe that have successfully replaced chairs with balls in classrooms to improve posture and reduce inactivity in young children. This practice is being slowly introduced into American schools through therapists treating children with special needs. Parents who are concerned about their children's posture have reported that requiring their children to sit on balls while watching television or playing video games is an effective way to encourage movement and exercise in otherwise inactive, kyphotic sitting postures.

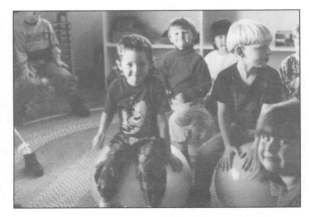

Ball Sizing Suggestions: *(based on twenty years of clinical experience)*

Person's Height	Ball Size		
Children 1-2 1/2 yrs	30cm	12	inches
Children 3-5 yrs	35cm	14	inches
5 yrs to 4'11" tall	45cm	18	inches
5' to 5'7"	55cm	21 1/2	inches
5'8" to 6'2"	65cm	25	inches
6'3" to 6'9"	75cm	29 1/2	inches
Over 6'10"	85cm	33 1/2	inches

The ball should be fitted appropriately to each person's body proportions so their hips and knees are bent at 90° angles [Klein-Vogelbach, Kucera]. If a person's height is between the specifications, they may need the larger size if they have long legs or carry extra weight for their height. If there is doubt, a larger ball is recommended because it can be slightly underinflated.

General Safety Instructions

1. Keep the ball away from sources of heat or direct sunlight for extended periods of time.

2. Check the area and clothing for sharp objects that may puncture the ball.

3. Provide enough unobstructed space so there is no furniture or other objects in the immediate area that could cause injury.

4. Maintain optimal posture when bouncing. **Do not combine bouncing with bending, twisting or rotating the spine.**

5. Do the exercises slowly and with control.

6. A heavy pony tail may cause discomfort to the neck. If so, modify this hair style.

7. Bare feet are recommended while exercising. However, if feet are slipping, rubber soled shoes are advised.

8. When wearing athletic shoes that have been worn outside, check the soles for pebbles. These may fall out of the soles and puncture the ball if it happens to roll over them.

9. Wear comfortable clothes that allow full range of movement. Denim jeans or tight fitting pants are usually too restrictive for exercises. Shorts should be at least knee length as bare skin will often stick to the ball, hinder movement and/or cause discomfort.

**Although therapists can increase their own exercise repertoire from this book, participant workshops and videos by qualified instructors are more effective mediums for mastering ball techniques. Just as ballet cannot be learned from a book, many therapeutic techniques, such as the Neuro-Developmental Treatment approach and manual therapy, must be learned from personal instruction. Therapists will gain a more thorough understanding of the exercises in an instructional setting where they practice being and/or treating different types of patients. The hands-on experience will then enable them to more safely and effectively guard and guide their patients through ball exercise programs. Videos also offer therapists the ability to review and practice techniques whenever necessary.

Suggested Sitting Position: Optimal Posture

Unfortunately, the running man of prehistoric times has become a sedentary modern man. Roughly 80% of the adult population in modernized countries will experience back pain in their life. Next to the common cold, it is the cause for the most absences from work costing billions of dollars a year and decreasing quality of life for millions of people. Scientific tests have proven that by changing one's behavior up to 70% of the costs of back pain can be avoided (Baviera, 1994).

Vertabrae

7 Cervical

12 Thoracic

5 Lumbar

5 Sacral (Sacrum)

4 Coccygeal (Coccyx)

In optimal posture, there are three dynamic curves of the spine. These curves combine with the disks between the vertebrae to absorb the forces of gravity through the spine in the most efficient manner. Studies show that the pressure on the disks in sitting is 30% greater than in standing. After ten years of age, the disks have no direct, internal blood supply and receive most of their nourishment through pressure changes created by movement of the spine. Lack of sufficient circulation to the disk leads to degeneration which can cause pain, stiffness and starts a vicious circle of inactivity and further damage.

In muscles, static work requires greater consumption of energy for smaller effort. Dynamic work increases the blood circulation up to twenty times that of static work and can be performed for a longer period without fatigue (Oliver and Middleditch, 1991). A larger base of support, i.e. sitting, creates more static positions and less muscle activity is required to maintain the position. When standing upright, our body weight is balanced over a small surface. While walking, the base of support is even smaller when weight is momentarily balanced on one leg and muscles are activated in dynamic patterns. General health can be improved by reducing the amount of time spent in static, sitting positions.

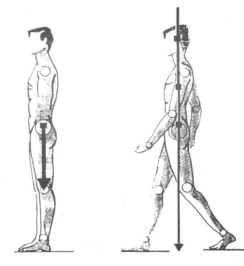

One tool to increase movement while sitting is the "Swiss Ball" because it is an unstable base of support which requires continual adjustments of the body to maintain balance. It is suggested that each person use a ball that is appropriately fitted to their body proportions to facilitate optimal posture (spinal alignment) and muscle balance. Ideally, the hips and knees of the person will be bent at 90° angles (Kucera, Klein-Vogelbach). The ball activates the muscles of the feet, legs, hips and spine in order to efficiently maintain the individual's balance (positioning their center of gravity over their base of support). For this reason, correct positioning is essential to ensure that muscles tighten properly to reinforce optimal joint alignment, posture and comfort. Using the wrong size ball cannot nly be uncomfortable and more difficult but may also be harmful by creating muscle imbalances and malalignment of the spine and joints (Refer to Ball Sizing Chart, page 26).

To Begin: Sit in the center of the ball with hips and knees bent at 90° angles and legs parallel at hips' width apart. Place feet firmly on the floor in proper alignment (avoid pronation or supination). Knees should be directly over ankles. In this position, ankles, knees and hips are centered. However, slouching is still possible. Use following methods to achieve optimal spinal alignment.

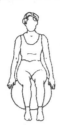

Notice: If hips are purposely positioned off-center, it takes more effort to balance and will become uncomfortable.

Methods to Achieve Optimal Posture:

Following are three methods to achieve optimal posture. The first two methods require conscious effort and verbal cues from an observer may be necessary to achieve correct alignment. In contrast, the third method facilitates optimal posture without conscious effort as the gentle compression and distraction caused by bouncing aligns the spine in its most efficient position independent of verbal cues and with consistent results.

1. Sit up as straight as possible by imagining puppet strings are attached to the top of head and are pulling up (Avoid pressing rib cage forward and arching lower back). Then, feel body weight drop into the ball. Relax shoulders and let arms hang at sides. Shoulders should be directly over hips and ears should be in line with shoulders (look in a mirror). If the spine is not properly aligned, use method #2 or #3.

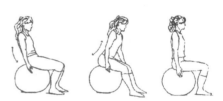

2. Let the ball roll forward until it touches the back of the legs allowing lower spine to curve. Then, roll the ball backward as far as possible allowing lower spine to arch. Now, find the position in between which is the most comfortable (symptom free or minimized symptom) and requires little effort. Tuck chin so ears are aligned over shoulders.

3. Begin with **Basic Bounce** by pressing feet into floor and tightening thigh and hip muscles to slightly lift trunk. Relax. Continue bouncing by alternately tightening and relaxing these muscles as vigorously as balance, coordination and comfort allow (See page 37). **Notice:** When bouncing, the spine will gravitate to the most comfortable, energy efficient position (optimal posture) by putting the body's center of gravity over its base of support to reduce any uneven compression or shearing forces between the vertebrae or stretch of ligaments or muscles. It will also activate the appropriate muscles automatically to support the spine in this posture.

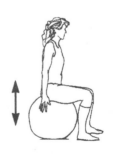

Maintain this posture when you stop bouncing.

Notice: Bounce and feel how abdominal muscles tighten. Now concentrate on relaxing the abdominal muscles while bouncing. Feel how difficult it is to do this and maintain the stability of the spine, especially while lifting feet one at a time.

CAUTION: **NEVER BEND OR TWIST SPINE WHILE BOUNCING AS THIS COULD CAUSE OR AGGRAVATE INJURY.**

Guarding Options for Therapists

Provide an unobstructed space for patient and therapist to exercise safely using the ball. Anyone who can walk unassisted or most people who use a cane for assistance should be capable of independently sitting on the ball and keeping their balance. If an ambulatory person still feels insecure exercising on the ball, take precautions to offer them a slight balance assist which can be either the light touch of another person or a stable object.

If the patient is exercising at home, instruct them to touch a chair, a wall or sofa placed at their side so they can release the object when they feel in control but can quickly touch it for balance. As soon as they feel comfortable without the assist, it is advisable to move away from the object. These patients can also use a Physio-Roll™ instead of a ball for less challenge.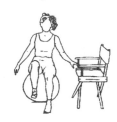

It is helpful to give the patient visual cues such as placing the patient in front of a mirror. The therapist can also increase the difficulty by removing visual cues. These techniques work well for both balls and the Physio-Roll™.

Patients who require an assistive device to walk or who are not ambulatory will need more guarding and hands-on control. If the patient is non-ambulatory, it may be safer to start them on a Physio-Roll™ which will be easier to control for both parties. If the therapist has to work hard to control the patient, either the exercise needs to be modified to a lower level of difficulty or the therapist should use techniques that increase their stability. Ideally, the patient should be working hard while the therapist should be *hardly* working.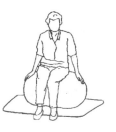

It is not effective for the therapist to sit on a chair to safely guard the patient at their waist because the therapist's spine will be in an uncomfortable and precarious position especially if the patient loses their balance. It is also not recommended for therapists to sit on a ball in front of the patient as it increases the risk of falling by putting both parties on an unstable base of support. There is a greater risk if the patient is touching the therapist for balance assistance. With the exception of standing behind the patient on a Physio-Roll™, guarding from behind is not efficient or safe. Only progress to sitting on a ball to demonstrate exercises once the patient does not require any guarding. Then, it can be a valuable method of instruction because it reduces treatment time required compared to sharing a ball. Also, people who are visual learners will perform better with visual instructions.

For both therapist and patient comfort, perform exercises on a mat or a well cushioned carpet. Following are suggestions for guarding techniques for patients who are cooperative and can follow directions, starting from most assistance and progressing to least assistance. Please practice these techniques with a partner before using them with a patient. **Remember the Physio-Roll and ball are unique tools because they offer an unstable base of support; therefore, there is always an element of risk involved.**

For complete control of the patients' balance when seated on the ball or Physio-Roll™:

The therapist should kneel on the floor in front of the patient. Place the patient's feet under therapist's calves. The therapist can lean their chest against the patient's knees and place their forearms on patient's thighs and their hands around patient's waist. Tell patient to rest their hands on the therapist's shoulders. **The patient should not be allowed to pull on therapist.**
From this position, the therapist can assist the patient with simple bouncing exercises (Chapter 1) or sitting spinal mobility exercises (Chapter 2).

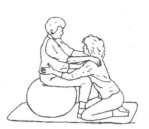

If the therapist is not comfortable sitting on heels:

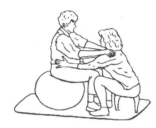

Sit on a low foot stool (so therapist can still use good body mechanics). The therapist can block the patient's feet with their arches and the patient's knees with their knees. The therapist should place their forearms on the patient's thighs and use their hands to control the patient's trunk from the waist. The patient can rest their hands on therapist's shoulders. **The patient should not be allowed to pull on therapist.**

Control from the waist:

Once a patient can balance their upper body without touching the therapist's shoulders, they can drop their hands to their sides. This will allow the patient to do any of the aerobic exercises using the upper extremities while the therapist can control them at the waist and legs.

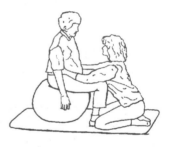

Control from knees:

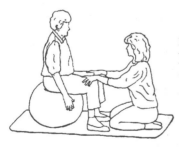

When the patient can control their pelvis, the therapist can move their hands down to the patient's thighs and then to their knees. Now, the patient can do any of the arm movements and will have to increase their participation in the bouncing while the therapist gives a more distal balance assist. If the patient starts to lose their balance, the therapist can quickly stabilize at the patient's waist or the patient can touch the therapist's shoulders. If the patient needs less assistance, the therapist can move their legs off the patient's feet but keep their hands on the patient's knees. The patient can then bounce from the ankles and perform some leg movements. However, if the patient starts to lose their balance, the therapist can reach in and stabilize their waist quickly. When patient no longer needs balance assistance, the therapist should remove their hands from the patient's knees but keep hands in close proximity to give stabilizing assistance when necessary.

Control for one sided weakness:

If a patient has only one-sided involvement, it is highly recommended to only assist the involved side. Follow previous directions for different levels of assistance. However, only stabilize the leg of the involved side between the therapist's legs. Instead of putting both hands around patient's waist, place one arm on top of patient's knee and one around waist. Patient can touch or rest their arm on the therapist's shoulder if necessary. If spasticity exists in the arm of involved side, other techniques can be used to control it. For example, using a therapeutic technique, place involved arm alongside of patient's body and, simultaneously, hold arm and waist. Of course, the degree of control can be modified by therapist's own expertise for each patient's individual needs.

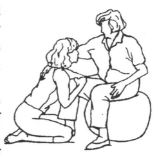

These techniques give balance and stability to the involved side while allowing the uninvolved side to participate freely and elicit automatic reactions for equilibrium and function on the involved side. Most of the aerobic exercises illustrated in Chapter 1 or sitting exercises in Chapter 2 can be modified for unilateral movement.

Transfers
To transfer a non-ambulatory patient on to a Physio-Roll™ from a sitting position.

Lift up patient's legs one at a time and roll the Physio-Roll™ under them until roll is against the chair or bed with both of the patient's legs resting on top of it *(1)*.

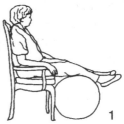

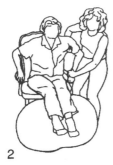

If the patient can push with their arms, they may be able to push out onto the roll independently. If the patient needs some assistance, the therapist can support the patient with one hand under their axilla and the other hand holding their forearm *(2)*.

Then the patient can roll out until their weight is on Physio-Roll™ and their feet drop down and touch the floor. Therapist needs to step forward as roll and patient move forward *(3)*. *Occasionally, the chair may tip forward as the patient begins to roll out, but it will fall back into place as the patient's weight is fully transferred.* The therapist can now follow the previous directions for guarding someone on the ball.

If the patient cannot help push with arms, it will require two people, one on each side, to support the patient and roll their body forward. Therapists can place one hand under each of the patient's axilla and support patient's forearm with other hand rolling patient forward in unison.

Exercising on a Physio-Roll™ (1)

The patient can also swivel their hips on the roll by moving one of their legs at a time *(2)* and letting their trunk turn so they are sitting on the end of the roll. Then, the therapist may sit behind them on the roll *(3)* and have many options for controlling the patient's trunk and arms while still having control of the roll with their legs*(4)*. If the patient cannot move their legs independently, the therapist can stand behind them for trunk support and help lift and move the legs one at a time. Otherwise, it may take two therapists, one standing behind patient for balance and one in front to move the legs.

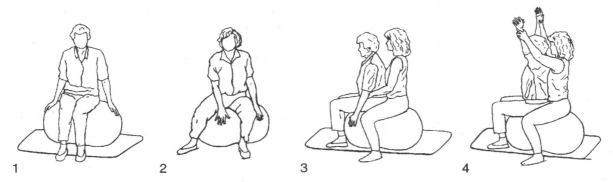

The therapist can also have the patient inch back to straddle the roll so they are sitting in the dip or saddle of the roll *(5)*. This helps control lower extremity adductor spasticity. It also allows the patient to put their hands on the roll in front of them giving them more security and balance assist *(6)*. In this position, there is little room for the therapist to sit on the roll behind the patient so they will need to use the previously mentioned front guarding techniques *(7)*.

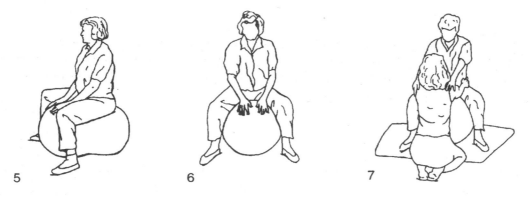

See transfer to side sit to help patient assume prone, supine or side lying positions over the roll. The Physio-Roll™ allows the patient to perform many of the other exercises shown in these positions with greater support and less difficulty. Assistance may still be required by a therapist.

Therapists may need to modify the guarding techniques to accommodate their own physical abilities, size and strength. There are many other simpler guarding methods that can be used as patients progress and need less assistance.

To transfer from Physio-Roll™ to floor:

Unlike a hard foam roll, the Physio-Roll™ is soft and molds to comfortably support the body as it moves. The Physio-Roll™ is a wonderful tool to safely transfer patients to and from the floor with minimal strength and risk on the part of the therapist(s). There are two basic ways this can be accomplished. Use previously mentioned method to transfer patient from chair to roll.

1. **From Physio-Roll™ to Long Sit:**
Stand behind the patient and place hands under patient's axilla from the front. Using proper body mechanics for hinging at the hips, be prepared to slowly bend forward. The patient should be instructed to walk their feet out and lean backward as their body rolls down the Physio-Roll™ toward the floor until their buttocks touch. The therapist can control speed at which patient descends from behind by using the leverage

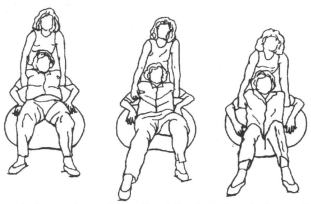

created as the patient leans backward and rests their trunk on the roll while their hands keep the patient's balance. If the patient cannot move their legs forward in a stepping pattern, an assistant will be needed to move feet.

    Reverse this process to transfer from floor to Physio-Roll™. The therapist may need to pull back slightly under patient's arms to start the roll moving as the patient leans backwards and lifts their hips by pushing their feet into the floor. While walking backward slowly, the therapist may need to help the patient come up to a seated position as their body rolls up onto the Physio-Roll™. Again, an assistant will be need to move the feet if the patient is unable.

2. **From Physio-Roll™ to Side Sit:** Stand behind the patient and place hands under patient's axilla from the front or back whichever is more comfortable. The patient should place both hands beside their hip on the roll. The patient should be instructed to walk feet out and slowly turn their body toward hands. The therapist can assist the patient in turning sideways on the roll as they slowly allow patient to lower sideways over the roll to the floor. The Physio-Roll™ will roll forward as the patient's body lowers to floor. The patient's lower arm should open out and allow the Physio-Roll™ to roll up under their axilla as the hips slowly lower to floor in side sitting position. I do not recommend this approach if the patient cannot assist with legs.

    Reverse this process to transfer from floor to sit. ***Caution: Do not start by putting patients axilla in the center of the roll because as they turn their hips will end up on the edge of the roll. Axilla needs to be placed towards the edge of the roll so hips will end in the center.***

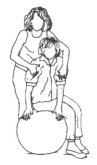 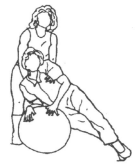 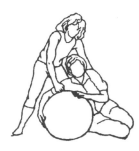

	Chapter 1	Cardiovascular Exercises

Date_____   Name_____

Basic Bounce   1:1

Starting Position: Sit correctly on the ball in optimal posture (see page 27).

Movement/Exercise: Begin bouncing by pushing feet into the floor and tightening thigh and hip muscles to slightly lift trunk, relax. Continue bouncing by alternating tightening and relaxing these muscles as vigorously as balance, coordination and comfort allow in optimal posture.

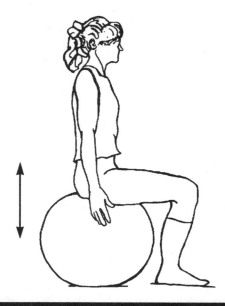

CAUTION: KEEP FEET PLANTED ON FLOOR. DO NOT BEND OR TWIST SPINE WHILE BOUNCING.

Breathing: Monitor heart rate. If winded, bounce less vigorously.

Modification: Lightly touch hands to ball or stable object for balance assistance.

Beats/min_____   **Repeat_____Times**

Do_____Times/day

Purpose/Goal_____

_____

Comments: *Bouncing on the ball helps to align spine in optimal posture and activates the muscles around spine to tighten and support it. Bouncing for extended periods can increase postural endurance for unsupported sitting and standing.*

Date_____   Name_____

Toe Raises with Bounce   1:2

Starting Position: Sit correctly on the ball in optimal posture.

Movement/Exercise: Begin bouncing by raising and lowering heels. Bounce as vigorously as comfort, balance and coordination allow.

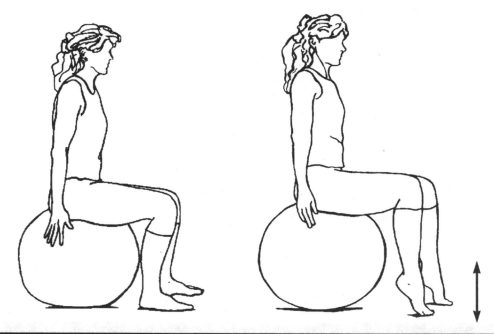

CAUTION: *KEEP TOES PLANTED ON FLOOR, WITH HIPS, KNEES AND FEET ALIGNED. DO NOT BEND OR TWIST SPINE WHILE BOUNCING.*

Breathing: Monitor heart rate. If winded, bounce less vigorously.

Modification: Lightly touch hands to ball or stable object for balance assistance.

Progression: Add light weights to wrists or hands.

Beats/min_____   /   Weights_____   /   Repeat____Times   /   Do____Times/day

Purpose/Goal_____

_____

Comments: *While the benefits for the spine are the same as in the Basic Bounce, this creates a different proprioceptive input for the knee and ankle. Momentum is initiated and absorbed by muscles around the ankle, rather than above the knee, gently training jumping and landing.*

Shoulder Shrug with Bounce 1:3

Starting Position: Sit correctly on ball in optimal posture.

Movement: Begin bouncing by raising and lowering shoulders. Bounce as vigorously as comfort, balance and coordination allow.

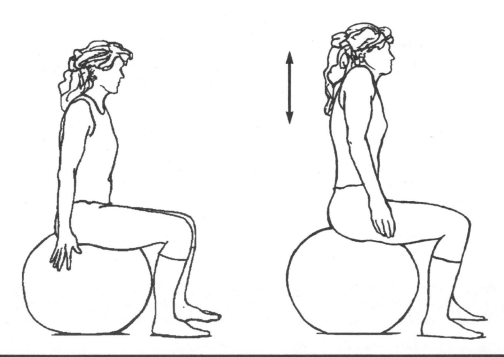

CAUTION: *KEEP FEET PLANTED ON FLOOR. DO NOT BEND OR TWIST SPINE WHILE BOUNCING. KEEP NECK STABLE.*

Breathing: Monitor heart rate. If winded, bounce less vigorously.

Progression: Add light weights to wrist or hands.

Beats/min_____ **Weights_____**

Repeat_____Times **Do_____Times/day**

Purpose/Goal:_____

_____

Comments: *Tight upper shoulder and neck muscles should relax while providing benefits mentioned in the Basic Bounce. Start gently if neck problems exist.*

© 1995 by Joanne Posner-Mayer, PT

Date_____   Name_____

Tight Arm Circles with Bounce   1:4

Starting Position: Sit correctly on ball in optimal posture. Raise straight arms out to side at shoulder level.

Movement: Keeping arms and wrists straight, draw large circles quickly with finger tips . (Body will bounce from the momentum produced by arms.) Rest. Reverse direction.

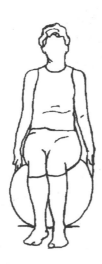 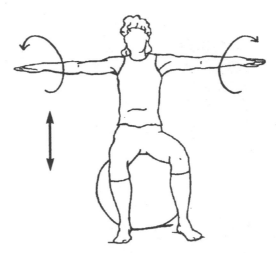

CAUTION: *KEEP FEET PLANTED ON FLOOR. DO NOT ALLOW SHOULDERS TO ELEVATE DURING EXERCISE.*

Breathing: Do not hold breath. Breathe comfortably.

Modification:
1. Move arms up and down in quick flutters.
2. Move arms forward and backward in quick flutters.
3. Lower arm height to comfort level.

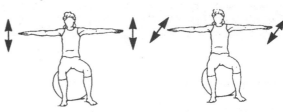

Progression:
1. Move arms in small circles (approximately 4 to 6 inches in diameter)
2. Flutter arms and *do not* allow the body to *bounce* on the ball. Absorb the momentum created by the arms.

Beats/min_____   /   Repeat_____Times   /   Do_____Times/day

Purpose/Goal _____

_____

Comments: *Feel how the muscles of the back and stomach tighten simultaneously to stabilize the spine as the arms move, especially when absorbing momentum to keep the body from bouncing.*

Drumming with Bounce   1:5

Starting Position: Sit correctly on ball in optimal posture.

Movement: Keeping wrists stiff, begin bouncing by raising and lowering forearms simultaneously as if hitting a drum.

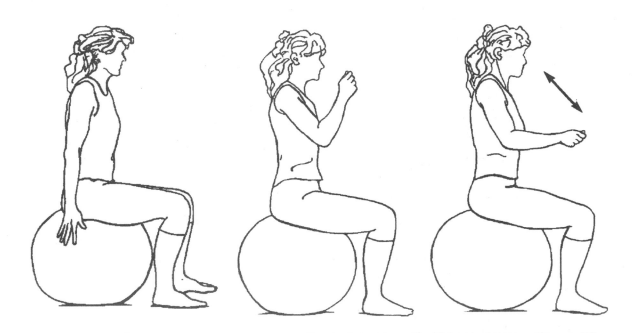

CAUTION: *KEEP FEET PLANTED ON FLOOR. KEEP HANDS AWAY FROM FACE.*

Breathing: Monitor heart rate. If winded, bounce less vigorously.

Progression:
1. Add light weights to wrist or hands.
2. Repeat movement but *do not* allow body to *bounce*. Notice how trunk muscles tighten to absorb the momentum.

Beats/min_____ / Weights_____ / Repeat_____Times / Do_____Times/day

Purpose/Goal:_____

_____

Comments: While providing the same benefits of the Basic Bounce, feel the difference in the spine and legs when more force is added to the up beat, then to the down beat compared to equal force in each direction.

Date_____ Name_____

Arm Swing with Bounce   1:6

Starting Position: Sit correctly on ball in optimal posture.

Movement: Place one arm forward and other arm backward. Switch arms in a swinging motion. Add bouncing in same tempo.

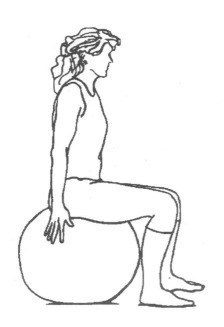
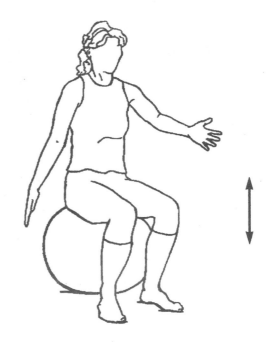

CAUTION: *KEEP FEET PLANTED ON FLOOR.*

Breathing: Monitor heart rate. If winded, bounce less vigorously.

Modification:
1. Only swing one arm at a time.
2. Touch ball or stable object with other hand for balance assistance.

Progression: Increase difficulty by swinging arms higher and/or increasing tempo (speed of bouncing and swinging). Add light weights to wrist or hands.

Beats/min_____   **Weights**_____

Repeat_____**Times**   **Do**_____**Times/day**

Purpose/Goal:_____

_____

Comments: By moving the arms, the balance and stability of the spine are further challenged and heart rate will also increase.

© 1995 by Joanne Posner-Mayer, PT

Date_____   Name_____

Front/Back Clap with Bounce   1:7

Starting Position: Sit correctly on ball in optimal posture.

Movement: Clap hands in front of body, then behind. Add bouncing in tempo.

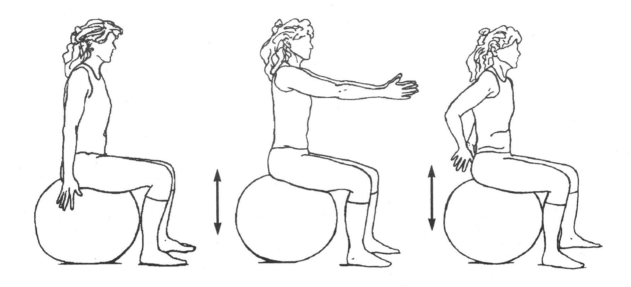

CAUTION: *KEEP FEET PLANTED ON FLOOR.*

Breathing: Monitor heart rate. If winded, bounce less vigorously.

Modification:
1. Only swing one arm at a time.
2. Touch ball or stable object with other hand for balance assistance.

Progression: Increase speed of arm swing, size of bounce and tempo of bounce.

Beats/min_____

Repeat_____Times

Do_____Times/day

Purpose/Goal:_____

_____

Comments: *By moving the arms, the stability of the spine is further challenged and heart rate will also increase. The arm movements, combined with the rhythmic bouncing and clapping, will challenge coordination, motor planning and balance.*

Date_____   Name_____

Overhead Clap with Bounce   1:8

Starting Position: Sit correctly on ball in optimal posture with fingers touching ball.

Movement: Clap hands over head then clap hands on the ball. Add bouncing in tempo.

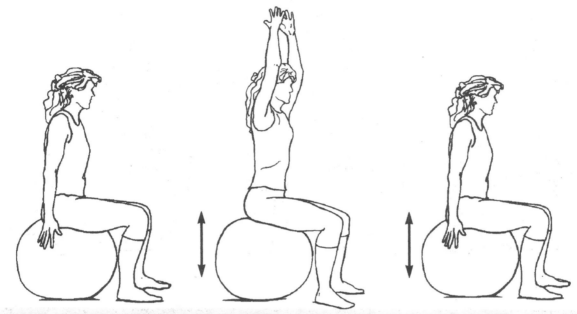

CAUTION: *KEEP FEET PLANTED ON FLOOR. KEEP SHOULDERS DOWN.*

Breathing: Monitor heart rate. If winded, bounce less vigorously.

Modification:
1. Raise arms slightly then lower and tap ball.
2. Raise arms and clap in front of body staying in pain free range. Lower and tap ball.

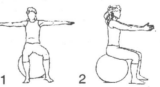

Progression: Increase speed of arm swing, size of bounce and tempo of bounce.

Beats/min_____   /   Repeat_____Times   /   Do_____Times/day

Purpose/Goal:_____

_____

Comments: By mobilizing the arms, the stability of the spine is further challenged and heart rate will also increase. The arm movements, combined with the rhythmic bouncing and clapping, will challenge coordination, motor planning and balance.

Shoulder Taps with Reach Out   1:9

Starting Position: Sit correctly on ball in optimal posture. Touch hands to shoulders with elbows out to side. Lift elbows out to shoulder height.

Movement: Reach hands out to side by straightening elbows. Return to starting position. Repeat. Add bouncing in tempo.

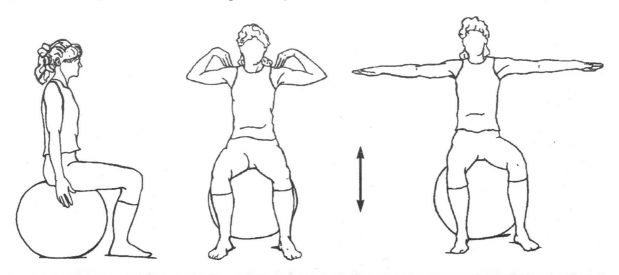

CAUTION: *KEEP FEET PLANTED ON FLOOR. KEEP SHOULDERS DOWN.*

Breathing: Monitor heart rate. If winded, bounce less vigorously.

Modification:
1. Reach out arms only as far as comfort allows.
2. Only reach out one arm at a time.
3. Touch ball or stable object with other hand for balance assistance.

Progression:
1. Increase speed of arm swing, size of bounce and tempo of bounce.
2. Add light weights to wrists or hands.

Beats/min_____   Weights_____

Repeat_____Times   Do_____Times/day

Purpose/Goal:_____

_____

Comments: By mobilizing the arms, the stability of the spine is further challenged and heart rate will also increase. The arm movements, combined with the rhythmic bouncing, will challenge coordination, motor planning and balance.

Shoulder Taps with Reach Up   1:10

Starting Position: Sit correctly on ball in optimal posture. Touch hands to shoulders and lift elbows to shoulder height.

Movement: Raise hands up toward ceiling as high as possible and then touch hands to shoulders. Add bouncing in tempo.

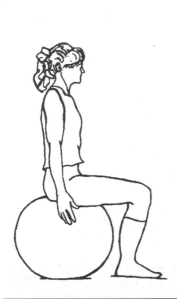 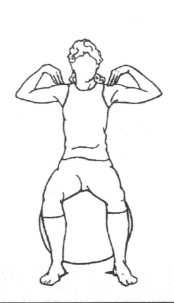 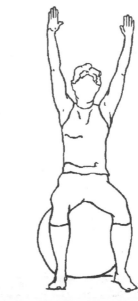

Breathing: Monitor heart rate. If winded, bounce less vigorously.

Modification:
1. Raise arms only as far as comfort allows.
2. Only raise one arm at a time.
3. Touch ball or stable object with other hand for balance assistance.

Progression:
1. Increase speed of arms, size of bounce and tempo of bounce.
2. Add light weights to wrist or hands.

Beats/min_____   Weights_____

Repeat_____Times   Do_____Times/day

Purpose/Goal:_____

_____

Comments: By moving the arms, the stability of the spine is further challenged and heart rate will also increase. The arm movements, combined with the rhythmic bouncing, will challenge coordination, motor planning and balance.

Date_____   Name_____

Asymmetrical Arms   *1:11*

Starting Position: Sit correctly on ball in optimal posture. Touch hands to shoulders with elbows out to side. Lift elbows to shoulder height.

Movement: Reach one arm up and one arm out. Return hands to shoulders and alternate sides. Add bouncing to tempo.

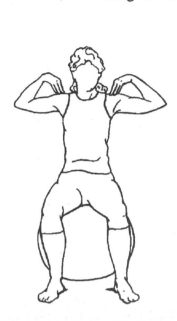
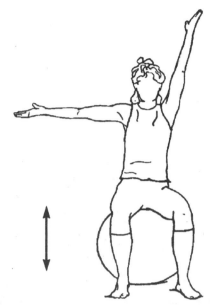

CAUTION: KEEP FEET PLANTED ON FLOOR. KEEP SHOULDERS DOWN.

Breathing: Monitor heart rate. If winded, bounce less vigorously.

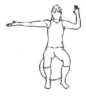

Modification: Reach arms only as far as comfort allows.

Progression:
1. Increase speed of arm swing, size of bounce and tempo of bounce.
2. Add light weights to wrists or hands.

Beats/min_____   Weights_____

Repeat_____Times   Do_____Times/day

Purpose/Goal:_____

_____

Comments: *Asymmetrical arm movements will add challenge to trunk stability, balance and coordination.*

Date_____   Name_____

Alternate "V" Arms   1:12

Starting Position: Sit correctly on ball in optimal posture. Raise arms overhead in a "V" position.

Movement: Let one elbow bend and drop towards center of chest as if arm is pulling an elastic cord. Return to start and alternate sides. Add bouncing in tempo.

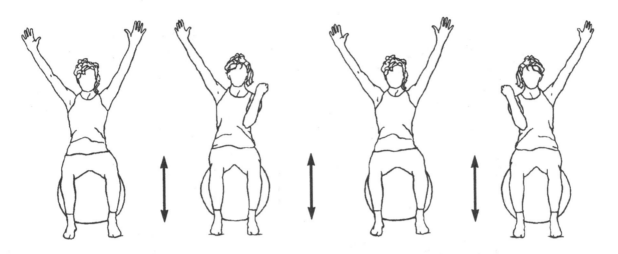

CAUTION: *KEEP FEET PLANTED ON FLOOR.*

Breathing: Monitor heart rate. If winded, bounce less vigorously.

Modification:
1. Only raise one arm at a time.
2. Touch ball or stable object with one hand for balance assistance.

Progression:
1. Increase speed of arm swing, size of bounce and tempo of bounce.
2. Add light weights to wrists or hands.

Beats/min_____   Weights_____

Repeat_____Times   Do_____Times/day

Purpose/Goal:_____

_____

Comments: Asymmetrical arm movements will add challenge to trunk stability, balance and coordination.

© 1995 by Joanne Posner-Mayer, PT

Date_____   Name_____

Arm Punches   *1:13*

Starting Position: Sit correctly on ball in optimal posture.

Movement: Many possibilities: punch alternate arms forward, punch alternate arms up, alternate punching one arm up and one arm across the chest. Add bouncing in tempo.

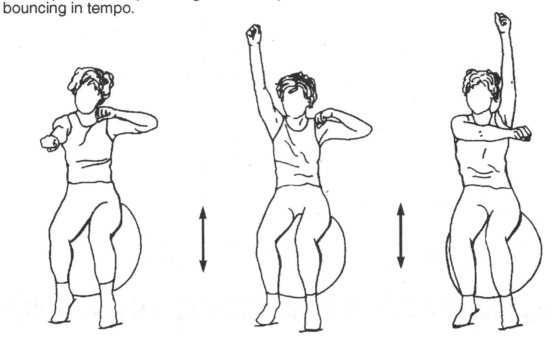

CAUTION: *KEEP FEET PLANTED ON FLOOR.*

Breathing: Monitor heart rate. If winded, bounce less vigorously.

Modification: Touch object for balance assistance. Only punch one arm at a time.

Progression: Add light weights to wrists or hands.

Beats/min_____   Weights_____

Repeat_____Times   Do_____Times/day

Purpose/Goal:_____
_____

Comments: *Many other arm movements can be created. Use imagination as the possibilities are limitless.*

Date_____ Name_____

Front Foot Tap 1:14

Starting Position: Sit correctly on ball in optimal posture. Begin Basic Bouncing.

Movement: With one bounce, tap one heel forward. With next bounce, bring foot back to start and alternate legs.

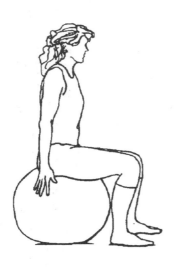 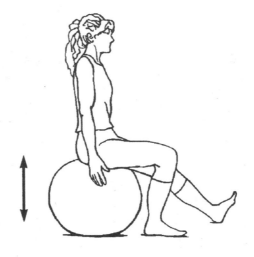

CAUTION: *MAKE SURE EXERCISE CAN BE DONE WITHOUT BOUNCING.*

Breathing: Monitor heart rate. If winded, bounce less vigorously.

Modification: Touch hands to ball or stable object for balance assistance.

Progression:
1. Initiate bounce by raising heels (see page 38).
2. Alternate legs with each bounce.
3. Add desired arm movement from previous section.

Beats/min_____

Repeat_____Times

Do_____Times/day

Purpose/Goal:_____

_____

Comments: *Moving the feet reduces the base of support and keeps the center of gravity changing. This forces the body to continually make unconscious/automatic adjustments to maintain balance.*

Side Foot Tap   *1:15*

Starting Position: Sit correctly on ball in optimal posture.   Position arms folded in front or as desired. Begin Basic Bouncing.

Movement: With one bounce, tap right foot to the right side. With next bounce, tap foot back to center. Repeat with left foot and alternate sides.

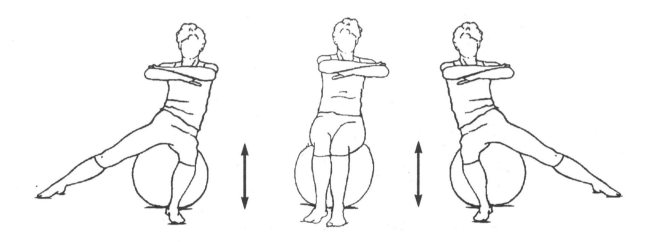

CAUTION: MAKE SURE EXERCISE CAN BE DONE WITHOUT BOUNCING.

Breathing: Monitor heart rate. If winded, bounce less vigorously.

Modification: Touch hands to ball or stable object for balance assistance.

Progression:
1. Initiate bounce by raising heels (see page 38).
2. Alternate legs with each bounce.
3. Add desired arm movement from previous exercises.

Beats/min_____

Repeat_____Times   Do_____Times/day

Purpose/Goal:_____

_____

Comments: Moving the feet reduces the base of support and keeps the center of gravity changing. This forces the body to continually make unconscious/automatic adjustments to maintain balance.

Date_____   Name_____

Leg March   1:16

Starting Position: Sit correctly on ball in optimal posture. Begin Basic Bouncing.
Position arms out to side or as desired.

Movement: With one bounce, lift one knee up. With next bounce, put foot down.
Repeat with other leg. Alternate sides.

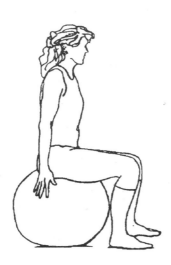
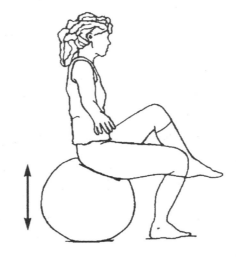

CAUTION: *MAKE SURE EXERCISE CAN BE DONE WITHOUT BOUNCING. DO
NOT ALLOW TRUNK TO BEND WHEN RAISING KNEE UP.*

Breathing: Monitor heart rate. If winded, bounce less vigorously.

Modification: Touch hands to ball or stable object for balance assist.

Progression:
1. Initiate bounce by raising heels (see page).
2. Alternate legs with each bounce.
3. Add desired arm movement from previous section.

Beats/min_____

Repeat_____Times   Do_____Times/day

Purpose/Goal:_____

_____

*Comments: Moving the feet reduces the base of support and keeps the center of gravity changing.
This forces the body to continually make unconscious/automatic adjustments to maintain balance.*

Kick Out   1:17

Starting Position: Sit correctly on ball in optimal posture. Begin Basic Bouncing. Position arms at sides or as desired.

Movement: With one bounce, kick foot up until knee is as straight as is comfortable (do not compensate by bending trunk). With next bounce, put foot down. Repeat with other leg. Alternate sides.

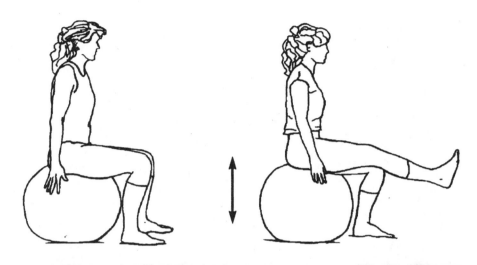

**CAUTION: MAKE SURE EXERCISE CAN BE DONE WITHOUT BOUNCING.
TIGHT HAMSTRINGS WILL NOT ALLOW KNEE TO STRAIGHTEN.**

Breathing: Monitor heart rate. If winded, bounce less vigorously.

Modification:
1. Touch hands to ball or stable object for balance assistance.
2. Lower leg height.

Progression:
1. Initiate bounce by raising heels (see page 38).
2. Alternate legs with each bounce.
3. Add desired arm movement from previous exercises.

Beats/min_____   /   Repeat_____Times   /   Do_____Times/day

Purpose/Goal:_____

_____

Comments: *Moving the feet reduces the base of support and keeps the center of gravity changing. This forces the body to continually make unconscious/automatic adjustments to maintain balance.*

Date_____   Name_____

Step Around Ball   *1:18*

Starting Position: Sit correctly on ball in optimal posture. Begin Basic Bouncing. Position arms at sides or as desired.

Movement: On upward half of bounce, step one foot sideways. With next bounce, bring other foot to meet it. Repeat and circle the ball. Alternate to other side.

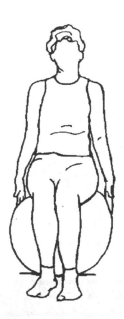 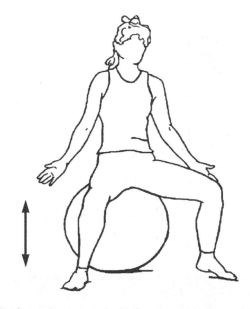

CAUTION: *MAKE SURE EXERCISE CAN BE DONE WITHOUT BOUNCING.*

Breathing: Monitor heart rate. If winded, bounce less vigorously.

Modification: Touch hands to ball or stable object for balance assistance.

Progression:
1. Initiate bounce by raising heels (see page 38).
2. Add desired arm movement from previous exercises.

Beats/min_____   /   **Repeat _____Times**   /   **Do_____Times/day**

Purpose/Goal:_____

_____

Comments: *Moving the feet reduces the base of support and keeps the center of gravity changing. This forces the body to continually make unconscious/automatic adjustments to maintain balance.*

Date_____   Name_____

Hop Around Ball

Starting Position: Sit correctly on ball in optimal posture. Begin Basic Bouncing. Position arms at sides or as desired.

Movement: With one bounce, hop both feet to side. Repeat hopping and circle the ball.

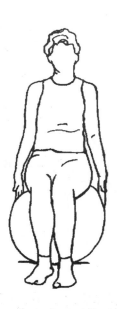 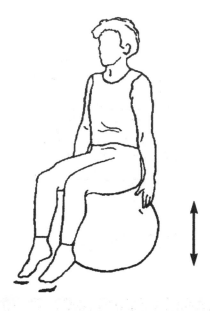

CAUTION: *MOVE BODY ON THE UPWARD HALF OF THE BOUNCE.*

Breathing: Monitor heart rate. If winded, bounce less vigorously.

Modification: Touch hands to ball for balance assist.

Progression: Add desired arm movement from previous section.

Beats/min_____

Repeat_____Times   Do_____Times/day

Purpose/Goal:_____

_____

Comments: Moving the feet reduces the base of support and keeps the center of gravity changing which forces the body to continually make unconscious/automatic adjustments to maintain balance. This is also a gentle way to train the body to decelerate impact on landing.

Date_____   Name_____

March-Arm and Leg   1:20

Starting Position: Sit correctly on ball in optimal posture. Begin Basic Bouncing.

Movement: With one bounce, swing one arm forward and lift opposite knee. With next bounce, return to start. Repeat to other side. Alternate.

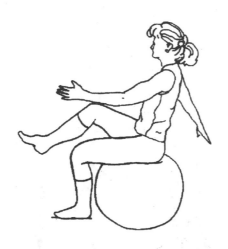 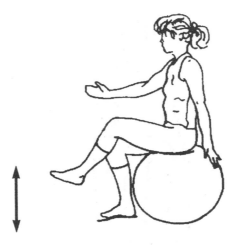

CAUTION: *ONLY PROGRESS TO THIS EXERCISE WHEN EXERCISES 1:6 AND 1:17 HAVE BEEN MASTERED.*

Breathing: Monitor heart rate. If winded, bounce less vigorously.

Modification: Tap one foot forward to touch the floor.

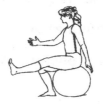

Progression:
1. Alternate opposite arms and legs with same bounce.
2. Kick foot until knee is straight (Tight hamstring muscles will not allow the knee to straighten).
3. Add light weights to wrists or hands.

Beats/min_____   /   Weights_____   /   Repeat_____Times   /   Do_____Times/day

Purpose/Goal:_____

_____

Comments: Moving the feet and arms at the same time requires more coordination and participation from muscles stabilizing the spine which are required to control the momentum and to automatically maintain the body's balance.

Date_____ Name_____

Unilateral Arms and Legs

Starting Position: Sit correctly on ball in optimal posture with arms relaxed at sides. Begin Basic Bouncing.

Movement: With one bounce, extend right leg forward and slightly out to side while lifting right arm up and slightly to side. With next bounce, return to start. Repeat to other side.

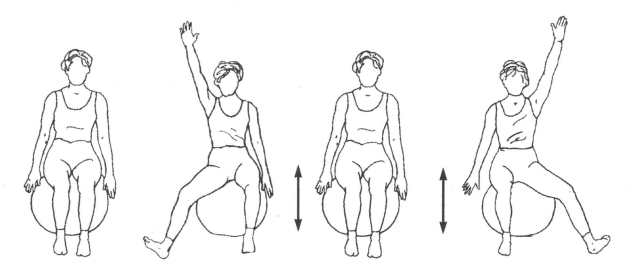

CAUTION: KEEP KNEES IN LINE WITH FEET.

Breathing: Monitor heart rate. If winded, bounce less vigorously.

Modification: Lift arms only as high as comfortable.

Progression:
1. Increase speed of arms and tempo of bounce and/or size of bounce.
2. Add light weight to wrists or hands.

Beats/min_____   **Weights_____**

Repeat_____Times   **Do_____Times/day**

Purpose/Goal:_____

_____

Comments: Moving the feet and arms at the same time requires more participation from muscles stabilizing the spine which are required to control the momentum and automatically maintain the body's balance as the center of gravity and support surface keeps changing.

Date_____   Name_____

Cossack Dance   1: 22

Starting Position: Sit correctly on ball in optimal posture. Raise arms straight in front at shoulder level. Begin Basic Bouncing.

Movement: With one bounce, extend right leg and right arm out to side and pull left hand into shoulder keeping elbow out to side at shoulder height. With next bounce, return to start. Repeat to other side.

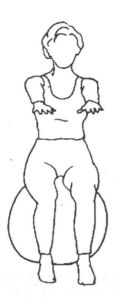 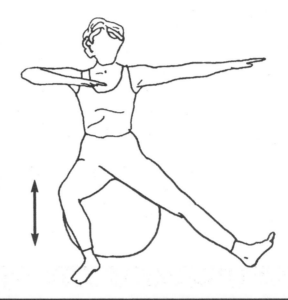

CAUTION: *KEEP KNEES IN LINE WITH FEET.*

Breathing: Monitor heart rate. If winded, bounce less vigorously.

Modification: Lift arms only as high as comfortable.

Progression:
1. Increase speed of arms and tempo of bounce and/or size of bounce.
2. Add light weights to wrist or hands.

Beats/min_____   Weights_____

Repeat_____Times   Do_____Times/day

Purpose/Goal:_____

_____

Comments: *Moving the feet and arms at the same time requires more participation from muscles stabilizing the spine which are required to control momentum and automatically maintain the body's balance as the center of gravity and support surface keeps changing.*

Date_____   Name_____

Half Jumping Jacks

Starting Position: Sit correctly on ball in optimal posture with arms relaxed at sides. Begin Basic Bouncing.

Movement: With one bounce, hop knees and feet apart and lift straight arms out level with shoulders. With next bounce, hop back to center and lower arms to sides.

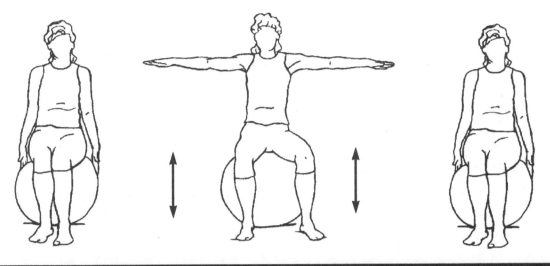

CAUTION: KEEP KNEES IN LINE WITH FEET.

Breathing: Monitor heart rate. If winded, bounce less vigorously.

Modification:
1. Move one leg and both arms. Switch legs.
2. Lift arms only as high as comfortable.

Progression:
1. Start with arms at shoulder level and lift above head as feet open.
2. Increase speed of arms and tempo of bounce and/or size of bounce.
3. Add light weights to wrists or hands.

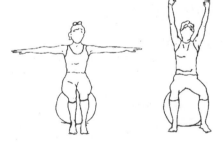

Beats/min_____ / Weights_____ / Repeat _____Times / Do_____Times/day

Purpose/Goal:_____

_____

Comments: Moving the feet and arms at the same time requires more participation from muscles stabilizing the spine which are required to control the momentum and automatically maintain the body's balance as the center of gravity and support surface keeps changing.

Full Jumping Jacks   *1:24*

Starting Position: Sit correctly on ball in optimal posture with arms relaxed at sides. Begin Basic Bouncing.

Movement: With one bounce, hop knees and feet apart and clap hands above head. With next bounce, hop back to center and clap hands to ball.

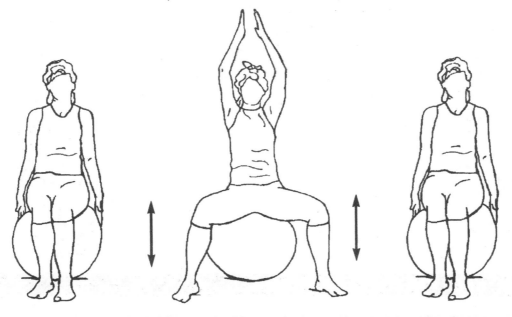

CAUTION: *KEEP KNEES IN LINE WITH FEET.*

Breathing: Monitor heart rate. If winded, bounce less vigorously.

Modification:
1. Move one leg and both arms. Switch legs.
2. Lift arms only as high as comfortable.

Progression:
1. Increase speed of arms and tempo of bounce and/or size of bounce.
2. Add light weights to wrist or hands.

Beats/min_____   /   Weights_____   /   Repeat_____Times   /   Do_____Times/day

Purpose/Goal:_____

_____

Comments: *Moving the feet and arms at the same time requires more participation from muscles stabilizing the spine which are required to control the momentum and automatically maintain the body's balance as the center of gravity and support surface keeps changing.*

Sitting Skier   *1:25*

Starting Position: Sit correctly on ball in optimal posture. With arms at sides, bend elbows slightly. Begin Basic Bouncing.

Movement: With each bounce, keep knees forward and, pivoting at the knee, hop feet equal distance from side to side. Arms swing in opposite direction from feet.

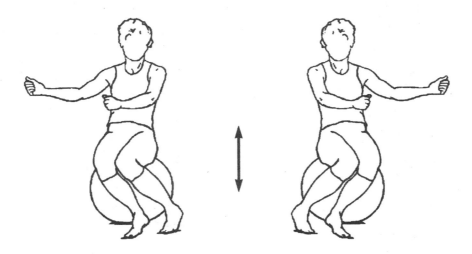

CAUTION: *KEEP TORSO STILL AND AVOID TWISTING OR BENDING SPINE.*

Breathing: Monitor heart rate. If winded, bounce less vigorously.

Modification: Move one leg and both arms. Switch legs.

Progression:
1. Increase speed of arms and legs and/or size of bounce.
2. Add light weights to wrist or hands.

Beats/min_____ / Weights_____ / Repeat_____Times / Do_____Times/day

Purpose/Goal:_____

_____

Comments: *Moving the feet and arms at the same time requires more participation from muscles stabilizing the spine which are required to control the momentum and to automatically maintain the body's balance.*

Arms and Legs In & Out   *1:26*

Starting Position: Sit correctly on ball in optimal posture. Lift elbows bent at right angles to shoulder level in front of body. Begin Basic Bouncing.

Movement: On one bounce, hop feet apart while opening and straightening arms out to sides. With next bounce, hop feet together and return to start. Repeat.

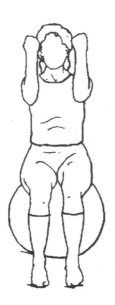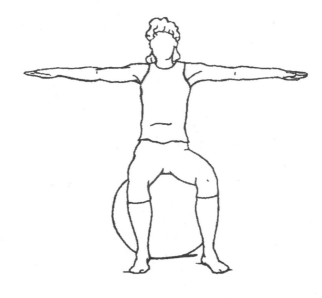

CAUTION: *KEEP KNEES IN LINE WITH FEET.*

Breathing: Monitor heart rate. If winded, bounce less vigorously.

Modification:
1. Move one leg and both arms. Switch legs.
2. Lift arms only as high as comfortable.

Progression:
1. Increase speed of arms and tempo of bounce and/or size of bounce.
2. Add light weights to wrist or hands.

Beats/min_____ / Weights_____ / Repeat_____Times / Do_____Times/day

Purpose/Goal:_____

_____

Comments: *Moving the feet and arms simultaneously requires more participation from muscles stabilizing the spine which are required to control the momentum and automatically maintain the body's balance as the center of gravity and support surface continually changes.*

Date_____   Name_____

Open and Close Around Ball   *1:27*

Starting Position: Sit correctly on ball in optimal posture (See page). Lift elbows bent at right angles to shoulder level in front of body. Begin Basic Bouncing.

Movement: On upward half of bounce, step one foot sideways and open arms out to sides. With next bounce, bring other foot to meet first foot and close arms. Repeat and circle ball. Alternate to other side.

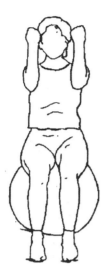 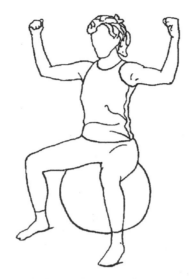 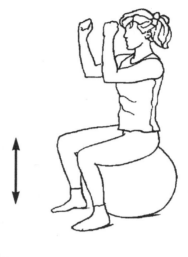

CAUTION: KEEP KNEES IN LINE WITH FEET.

Breathing: Monitor heart rate. If winded, bounce less vigorously.

Modification:
1. Move one leg and both arms, switch legs and do not travel in a circle.
2. Lift arms only as high as comfortable.

Progression:
1. Increase speed of arms and tempo of bounce and/or size of bounce.
2. Add light weights to wrist or hands.

Beats/min_____ / **Weights_____** / **Repeat____Times** / **Do_____Times/day**

Purpose/Goal:_____

_____

Comments: *Moving the feet and arms simultaneously requires more participation from muscles stabilizing the spine which are required to control the momentum and automatically maintain the body's balance as center of gravity and support surface continually changes.*

Chapter 2 — Spinal Mobility

Date_____ Name_____

Side to Side Hip Roll   2:1

Starting Position: Sit correctly on the ball in optimal posture.

Movement/Exercise: Using hips, gently roll ball from side to side as far as possible allowing ankles and knees to participate in the movement. Keep shoulders level.

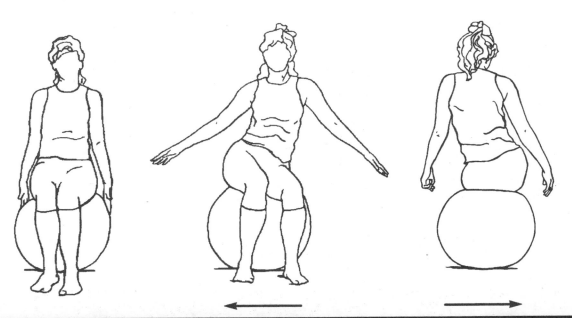

CAUTION: DO NOT FORCE MOVEMENTS SO THERE IS DISCOMFORT. STAY IN PAIN FREE RANGE.

Modification: Lightly touch hands to ball or stable object for balance assistance.

Progression: Feel the point where balance is challenged and hold for five seconds. Return to start.

Repeat_____ Times

Do_____Times/day

Purpose/ Goal:_____

_____

Comments: Notice if movement is equal to both sides. Movement restrictions could be caused by many factors. This exercise can gently mobilize the spine in side bending and expand the ribs. It can be a gentle range of motion and proprioceptive exercise for the hips, knees and ankles. This exercise can also be used effectively for improving balance skills.

Date_____   Name_____

Front and Back Hip Roll   2:2

Starting Position: Sit correctly on the ball in optimal posture.

Movement/Exercise: Roll ball forward and backward as far as possible using hips and allowing knees and ankles to participate in movement. Keep feet planted and allow lower spine to curve and arch.

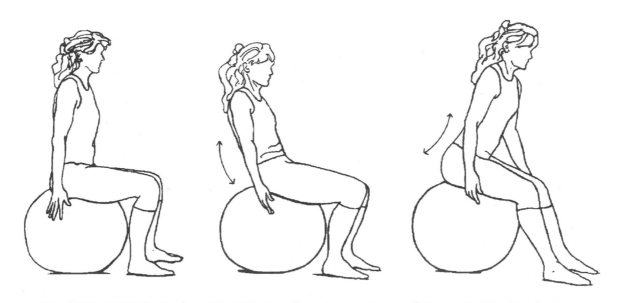

CAUTION: *DO NOT FORCE MOVEMENTS SO THERE IS DISCOMFORT. STAY IN PAIN FREE RANGE.*

Breathing: Inhale while rolling backward, exhale while rolling forward.

Modification: Lightly touch hands to ball or stable object for balance assistance.

Progression: Feel the point where balance is challenged and hold for five seconds. Return to start.

Repeat_____ Times

Do_____Times/day

Purpose/ Goal:_____

_____

Comments: *This exercise gently mobilizes the spine in flexion and extension. This is a gentle range of motion and proprioceptive exercise for the hips, knees and ankles. This exercise can also effectively be used for improving balance skills.*

Date_____   Name_____

Circular Hip Roll   2:3

Starting Position: Sit correctly on the ball in optimal posture. Be able to perform exercises 2:1 & 2:2.

Movement/Exercise: Move ball in a circle using hips (as if spinning a hula hoop) and allow knees and ankles to participate in the movement. Keep shoulders level and feet planted. Allow lower spine to move as much as possible. Rest. Reverse directions.

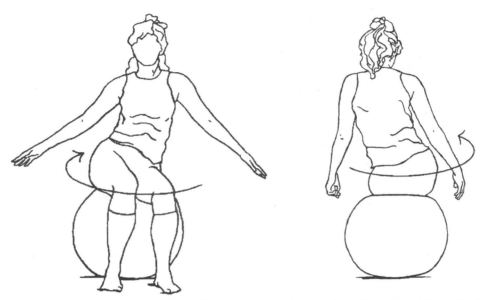

CAUTION: *KEEP FEET PLANTED ON THE FLOOR. STAY IN PAIN FREE RANGE.*

Modification: Lightly touch hands to ball or stable object for balance assistance.

Progression:
1. Enlarge the circle as much as possible without losing balance.
2. Allow body and shoulders to lean in opposite direction of hips while circling.

Repeat_____Times to Right   /   Repeat_____ Times to Left   /   Do_____Times/day

Purpose/ Goal:_____

_____

Comments: *This exercise gently mobilizes the spine in all directions. Notice if circle is asymmetrical or easier in one direction than the other. Movement restrictions could be caused by many factors. This is a gentle range of motion and proprioceptive exercise for the lower spine, hips, knees and ankles. It can be used for effectively improving balance skills.*

Date_____   Name_____

Gentle Trunk Rotation-Sitting 2:4

Starting Position: Sit correctly on the ball in optimal posture. Lift straight arms forward to shoulder level. Keep feet planted on floor and knees forward.

Movement/Exercise: Swing arms around behind body as far as possible allowing trunk, shoulders and head to turn in the same direction. Return to start and repeat in other direction. Ball should remain almost still during movement.

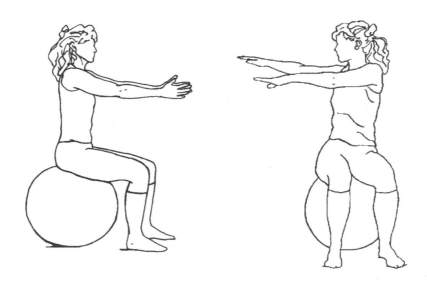

CAUTION: *DO NOT FORCE MOVEMENTS SO THERE IS DISCOMFORT. STAY IN PAIN FREE RANGE. SLOW DOWN MOTION IF BECOMING DIZZY.*

Breathing: Inhale on twist, exhale on return.

Modification: Move arms as far as comfort will allow.

Progression: Hold a medicine *(weighted)* ball or weights in hands to add momentum.

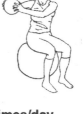

Hold ____Seconds / Weights_____ / Repeat_____ Times / Do_____Times/day

Purpose/ Goal:_____

_____

Comments: *This exercise gently mobilizes the spine in rotation. Notice if movement is equal to both sides. Movement restrictions could be caused by many factors in hips, spine and shoulders. This exercise gently mobilizes the spine and can also be used effectively for improving balance skills.*

© 1995 by Joanne Posner-Mayer, PT

Date_____   Name_____

Advanced Trunk Rotation-Sitting   2:5

Starting Position: Sit correctly on the ball in optimal posture. Raise straight arms forward to shoulder level. Spread feet as wide as comfort allows and keep knees over ankles.

Movement/Exercise: Reach arms sideways around body as far as possible allowing legs and body to turn in same direction. Keep knees in line with feet and straighten the back leg by raising back heel. Hold. Return to start and repeat in other direction. Ball should remain almost still during movement.

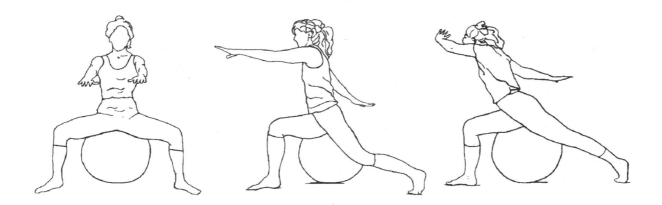

CAUTION: DO NOT FORCE MOVEMENTS SO THERE IS DISCOMFORT. SLOW DOWN MOTION IF BECOMING DIZZY.

Breathing: Do not hold breath. Breathe comfortably.

Modification: Move arms and straighten back leg as far as comfort will allow.

Hold_____Seconds   /   Repeat_____ Times   /   Do_____Times/day

Purpose/ Goal:_____

_____

Comments: *This exercise mobilizes the spine in rotation while stretching soft tissue from the toes of the back foot to the fingertips. Notice if movement is equal to both sides. Movement restrictions could be caused by many factors in lower extremities, spine and shoulders. This exercise can also be used effectively for improving balance skills and stretching tight hip flexor muscles.*

© 1995 by Joanne Posner-Mayer, PT

Supine Trunk Rotation   2:6

Starting Position: Lie on back with knees bent and feet on floor. Pick up ball with both hands and lift it above body.

Movement/Exercise: Keeping hands above head, simultaneously lower ball to the right as knees lower to the left. To reverse, tighten abdominal muscles and press lower back into floor before lifting ball and knees back to center. Repeat to other side.

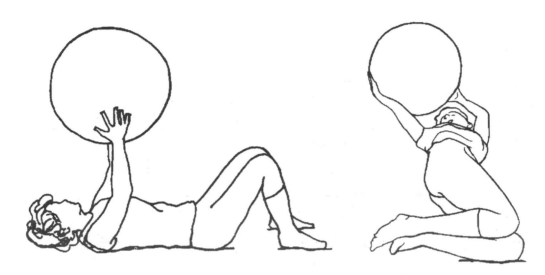

CAUTION: *STAY WITHIN PAIN FREE RANGE. DO NOT ALLOW LOWER BACK TO ARCH AS LEGS AND BALL ARE LIFTED AND LOWERED.*

Breathing: Inhale as ball is lowered, exhale on return.

Modification: Only move arms or legs.

Progression:
1. Lift weighted ball.
2. Increase tempo.
3. Straighten knee of top leg to increase stretch.

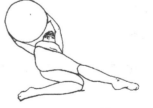

Hold_____Seconds / Weights_____ / Repeat_____Times / Do_____Times/day

Purpose/ Goal:_____

_____

Comments: *Feel how this stretches the soft tissue of the trunk diagonally from the lower hip to opposite shoulder as legs and ball lower. As legs lift, feel abdominal and chest muscles activate. Notice if movement is equal to both sides.*

© 1995 by Joanne Posner-Mayer, PT

Date_____   Name _____

Prone Rocking   2:7

Starting Position: Kneel behind ball and lie trunk over top of ball. Fold hands and place them on the ball. Relax neck and put head on ball.

Movement/Exercise: Dig toes into floor or place feet against wall. Straighten and bend knees to gently rock body forward and backward over ball. Allow head to hang.

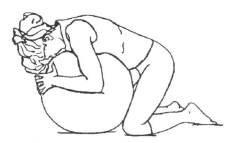 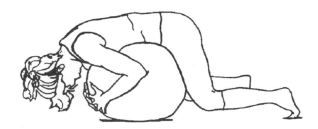

CAUTION: *STAY WITHIN PAIN FREE RANGE. DO NOT LET BALL ROLL OVER HANDS OR LONG HAIR.*

Breathing: Inhale while rolling forward, exhale on return. Focus on breathing into the back of the rib cage.

Modification: Touch hands to floor (out of the ball's path).

Progression:
1. Rock to side to side.
2. Roll ball underneath body in small circle by placing hands on floor and pushing on each extremity in sequence.

Hold____Seconds

Repeat_____ Times

Do_____Times/day

Purpose/ Goal:_____

_____

Comments: *Notice that there is a slight unweighting distraction of the vertebrae of the cervical spine as the muscles relax and head hangs. The farther the rock forward, the lower the distraction (reaching the upper thoracic vertebrae). On return, feel the weight loading each vertebra. There may be visible stiffness in the movement if there is restriction between vertebral segments.*

Date_____   Name_____

Kneel and Bow   *2:8*

Starting Position: Sit on heels with hands on top of ball. Lean forward letting the ball roll forward and relax spine into a C curve.

Movement/Exercise: Walk hands out and roll ball forward while slightly lifting buttocks. Relax spine and allow it to hang from shoulders and hips (like going under a limbo stick. Do not arch back like a cat). Go out as far as comfortable. Pause. Return to beginning curved position by lowering hips and rolling ball backward. Keep head between arms and eyes focused on floor.

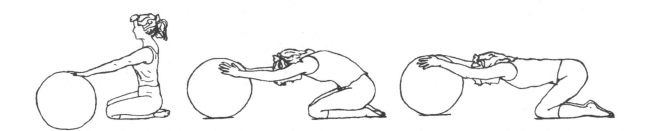

CAUTION: STAY WITHIN PAIN FREE RANGE. PAD KNEES IF NECESSARY.

Breathing: Inhale on roll out, exhale on return.

Modification:
1. If there is discomfort in shoulders, bend elbows out to side.
2. If unable to sit on heels, start exercise in kneeling position.
3. Sit in chair with ball in front on bed.

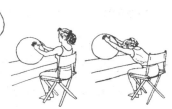

Progression: At end of stretch, shift weight back slightly, so that one hand can be pressed into the ball and lift the other hand off the ball one inch. As arm lifts, tighten abdominals and keep back flat.

Hold_____Seconds   Repeat _____ Times

Do_____Times/day

Purpose/ Goal:_____

_____

Comments: *Move slowly and try to feel each vertebra glide forward in succession starting at the neck as spine is extended . On return, try to feel each vertebra move backward in succession as spine is flexed. There will be visible stiffness in the movement of the spine if there is restriction between two or more vertebrae. This is also a gentle self controlled stretch for shoulder flexion.*

Date_____ Name_____

Kneel, Bow and Side Bend

Starting Position: Sit on heels with hands on top of ball. Lean forward letting the ball roll and relax spine into a C curve.

Movement/Exercise: Keeping hands still on ball and head between arms, roll ball to one side allowing trunk to turn. Hold and look under arm. Return to center and repeat to other side.

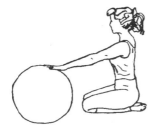
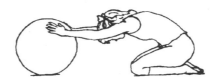
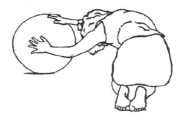

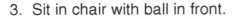

CAUTION: STAY WITHIN PAIN FREE RANGE. PAD KNEES IF NECESSARY.

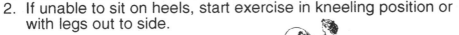

Breathing: Inhale on roll to side, exhale on return to center.

Modification:
1. If there is discomfort in shoulders, bend elbows out to side.
2. If unable to sit on heels, start exercise in kneeling position or with legs out to side.

3. Sit in chair with ball in front.

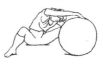

Progression: Make sure there is sufficient padding under knees. Roll out farther and lift feet from floor to balance weight on knees and hands. Begin exercise. Allow feet to sway from side to side to counter balance arms. Feel how this allows greater spinal rotation and rib expansion to each side.

Hold _____Seconds / Repeat _____ Times / Do_____Times/day

Purpose/ Goal:_____

_____

Comments: *Notice how ribs expand during lateral flexion on one side as the shoulder and hips get closer together on the other. There may be visible stiffness in the curve of the spine if there is restriction in the movement between two or more vertebrae. This exercise also allows gentle shoulder flexion plus internal and external rotation.*

Date_____ **Name**_____

Side Stretch 2:10

Starting Position: Kneel next to ball. Place top leg out to side and hands on ball.

Movement/Exercise: Press foot into floor and extend top leg allowing trunk to roll over ball sideways. Bring top arm up next to ear and let hand dangle towards floor increasing the stretch. Gently rock at end range. Return to start. Switch sides.

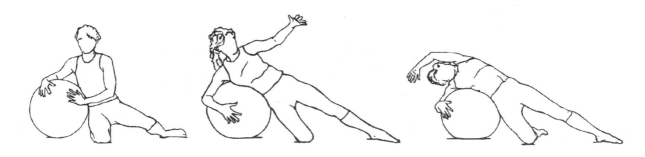

CAUTION: STAY WITHIN PAIN FREE RANGE.

Breathing: Inhale on stretch out, exhale when returning to start.

Modification:
1. Touch floor with top hand for balance.
2. Support head with lower hand.
3. Sit in chair or next to bed and use a smaller ball to roll.

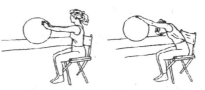

Progression: To increase stretch, push toes of *lower* leg into floor and extend knee to lie farther over ball.

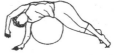

Hold_____**Seconds** / **Repeat**_____ **Times** / **Do**_____**Times/day**

Purpose/ Goal:_____

_____

Comments: *Feel how gravity assists in expanding ribs and the distance between ribs and hips as spine is gently mobilized laterally. One can do deep breathing exercises for various lobes of the lung as they pass over the top of the ball or self percussion using the hand of the lower arm.*

Date_____   Name_____

Trunk Rotation Stretch   2:11

Starting Position: Kneel next to ball. Rest upper torso and head sideways on ball with one arm on floor.

Movement/Exercise: Push with both legs allowing upper leg to extend as ball rolls under back. Free arm is brought up and out to side in a diagonal opening chest so that it is facing ceiling. Hips will turn slightly to follow trunk.

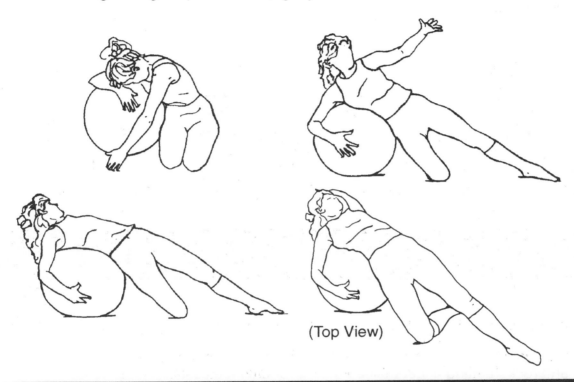

(Top View)

CAUTION: ONLY TURN AS FAR AS IS COMFORTABLE.

Breathing: Inhale while stretching, exhale while returning to start.

Modification: Support head with hand or touch lower hand to floor for balance assist.

Hold_____Seconds   /   Repeat_____Times   /   Do_____Times/day

Purpose/ Goal:_____

_____

Comments: *Feel how gravity helps in expanding the ribs and the distance between the lower hip and upper shoulder. Soft tissue can stretch as spine is gently mobilized in rotation while ball supports weight of the body.*

Date_____ Name_____

Squat and Rock 2:12

Starting Position: Sit on the ball. Walk feet forward while leaning trunk backward allowing ball to roll under mid-back.

Movement/Exercise: Bend at knees and hips and lower body into squat position (stay in pain free range). Press feet into floor while straightening and bending knees. Rock body backward and forward (to mid-back) on the ball. Only go as far as is comfortable.

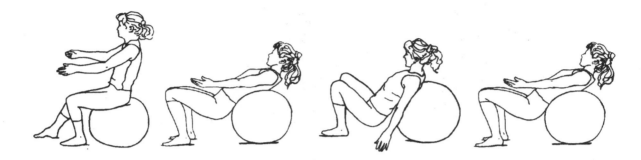

CAUTION: *IF DIZZY, TUCK CHIN. PREVENT FEET FROM SLIPPING BY PLACING TOES AGAINST STABLE OBJECT OR WEARING RUBBER SOLED SHOES. IF NECK MUSCLES FATIGUE, PLACE HANDS LIGHTLY BEHIND HEAD TO SUPPORT.*

Breathing: Inhale while rocking backward, exhale while rocking forward.

Modification: Let hands touch ball until in squat position then touch floor and rock. Letting fingers glide on floor for balance assist.

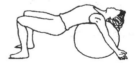

Progression: Let one or both hands glide on floor out to side to increase stretch of anterior chest and forearms. Straighten fingers out to increase forearm stretch.

Hold_____Seconds / Repeat_____ Times / Do_____Times/day

Purpose/ Goal:_____

_____

Comments: *Feel how gravity assists in expanding chest and ribs as spine is supported and gently mobilized into extension. (This exercise counteracts a rounded shoulder/forward head posture.) This is also a good proprioceptive exercise for hips, knees and ankles.*

© 1995 by Joanne Posner-Mayer, PT

Squat and Arch-Supported Extension 2:13

Starting Position: Assume Squat and Rock position (see page 12). Stay in pain free range.

Movement/Exercise: Reach arms overhead while straightening knees. Letting ball roll back as spine arches over ball. Reach for the floor with hand as far as is comfortable.

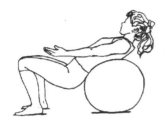 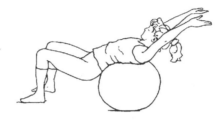 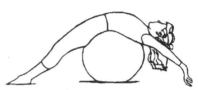

CAUTION: IF DIZZY, TUCK CHIN. PREVENT FEET FROM SLIPPING BY PLACING TOES AGAINST STABLE OBJECT OR WEARING RUBBER SOLED SHOES.

Breathing: Inhale on rock backward, exhale on rock forward.

Modification:
1. Let hands touch ball until in squat position then touch floor and rock backwards, letting fingers glide on floor for balance assist.
2. Place one hand behind head to support head and neck.

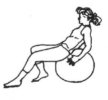

Hold _____Seconds

Repeat_____ Times

Do_____Times/day

Purpose/ Goal:_____

_____

Comments: *Feel how gravity assists in expanding chest and ribs as spine is gently mobilized into extension while fully supported by the ball. (This exercise counteracts a rounded shoulder/forward head posture.) This is also a good proprioceptive exercise for hips, knees and ankles while elongating hip flexors and shoulder flexors and abductors at end range.*

Chapter 3 Spinal Extension

Date_____   Name_____

Arm & Leg Lifts Quadruped   3:1

Starting Position: Kneel behind ball. Rest trunk over ball and put hands on floor under shoulders.

Movement/Exercise: Raise one arm and opposite leg squeezing the buttocks as leg lifts off floor. Return to start. Alternate to other side.

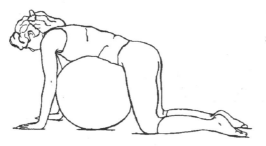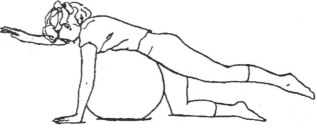

CAUTION: *STAY WITHIN PAIN FREE RANGE. AVOID ARCHING BACK BY KEEPING HIPS ON BALL WITH FACE PARALLEL TO FLOOR.*

Breathing: Inhale as leg lifts, exhale as leg lowers.

Modification:
1. Lift only one arm or leg at a time.
2. Place ball forward to support chin if unable to comfortably hold head up.

Progression:
1. Use cuff weights or resistive band on legs and/or arms.
2. Have an assistant give manual resistance as instructed by therapist (use either hold/relax or contract/relax techniques).

Hold_____Seconds   Weights_____

Repeat_____ Times   Do_____Times/day

Purpose/ Goal:_____

_____

Comments: The support of the ball takes pressure off the knees and wrists while the exercise gently tightens spinal extensor muscles as opposite arms and legs are lifting.

Date_____   Name_____

Gentle Upper Spine Extension-Prone   3:2

Starting Position: Kneel behind ball. Rest trunk over ball and place hands lightly behind head. Do not press on neck. Lower head and neck.

Movement/Exercise: Raise head, neck and upper back until head and arms are parallel to floor (keep elbows even with ears). Slowly lower and repeat.

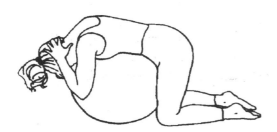 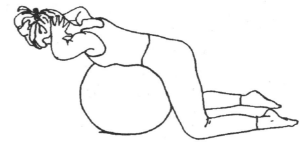

CAUTION: *STAY WITHIN PAIN FREE RANGE. AVOID ARCHING BACK OR NECK BY KEEPING LOWER RIBS ON BALL.*

Breathing: Inhale while lifting, exhale while lowering.

Modification: Lift only as far as comfort and/or strength allows.

Progression: Dig toes into floor and extend knees. Lift and lower as above.

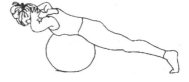

Hold_____Seconds

Repeat_____ Times

Do_____Times/day

Purpose/ Goal:_____

_____

Comments: *This exercise strengthens the entire back while keeping the lumbar spine unweighted and in optimal posture.*

© 1995 by Joanne Posner-Mayer, PT

Date_____   Name_____

Basic Push-Up   3:3

Starting Position: Kneel behind ball. Rest trunk over ball and put hands under shoulders. Dig toes into floor.

Movement/Exercise: Let ball roll as arms and legs straighten. Extend spine as far as is comfortable. Press hips into ball squeezing buttocks and tightening abdominals. Slowly lower to starting position.

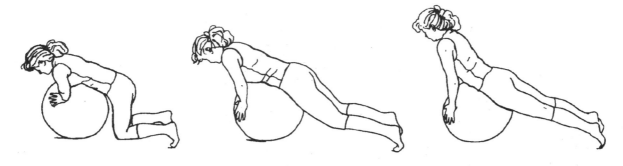

CAUTION: *STAY WITHIN PAIN FREE RANGE. KEEP NECK IN OPTIMAL POSITION.*

Breathing: Inhale while lifting, exhale while lowering.

Modification: As legs extend, do not fully extend spine by keeping elbows slightly bent or placing hands on the floor.

Progression:
1. Pick one leg up off floor. Balance and return foot to floor. Switch legs.
2. Pick up one leg and write alphabet in the air as big and fast as possible. Lower to floor. Switch legs.

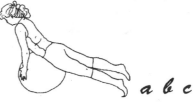

Hold_____Seconds

Repeat _____ Times

Do_____Times/day

Purpose/ Goal:_____

_____

Comments: *Feel the tightening of spinal extensors, flexors and shoulder girdle muscles. Lifting one leg changes the center of gravity and lessens the base of support. This challenges balance reactions and trains trunk stability while allowing for mobility of the leg.*

Airplane 3:4

Starting Position: Kneel behind ball. Rest trunk over ball and dig toes into floor. Raise arms out to side.

Movement/Exercise: Let ball roll down body while legs straighten. Lift trunk off ball as far as balance and comfort allow. Press hips into ball and squeeze buttocks. Slowly reverse and return to starting position.

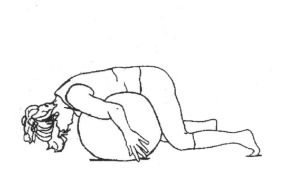 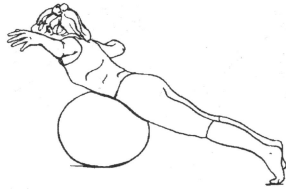

CAUTION: *STAY WITHIN PAIN FREE RANGE. KEEP NECK IN OPTIMAL POSITION.*

Breathing: Inhale when lifting, exhale when lowering.

Modification: Straighten legs and lift arms and trunk only as far as comfort allows.

Progression:
1. Pick one leg up off floor. Balance and return foot to floor. Alternate sides.
2. Pick up one leg and write alphabet in the air as big and fast as possible.
3. Use weights or resistive band in hands and/or on ankles.

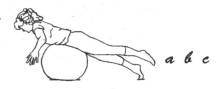

Hold_____Seconds   Weights _____

Repeat_____ Times   Do_____Times/day

Purpose/ Goal:_____

_____

Comments: *While this exercise targets the back muscles, notice the abdominal muscles tightening to support the weight of the body on the ball. Lifting one leg decreases the base of support and changes the center of gravity to challenge balance reactions. Moving the leg also trains trunk stability while allowing for mobility of the arms and legs.*

Date_____   Name_____

Hip Lift-Spinal Mobility   *3:5*

Starting Position: Lie on back. Place calves on ball and hands on floor at side. Press arms into floor and lift buttocks up until body is in a straight line.

Movement/Exercise: Lower to floor by rolling spine down one vertebra at a time. Reverse and curl spine up one vertebra at a time. Distance between hip bones and lowest rib decreases as the body is lifted and the spine is curled.

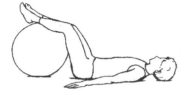 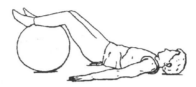 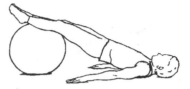

CAUTION: *STAY WITHIN PAIN FREE RANGE. DO NOT ARCH BACK.*

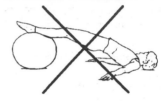

Breathing: Inhale when lifting, exhale when lowering.

Modification:
1. Lift only as far as comfort and balance allow.
2. Place ball closer to buttocks.

Progression:
1. Place ball farther down legs toward heels.
2. Pick one leg up off ball. Balance, lower leg onto ball. Alternate sides.
3. Pick one leg up and write alphabet in the air as big and fast as possible.
4. Add cuff weights at ankles.

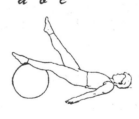

Hold_____Seconds / Weights_____ / Repeat_____ Times / Do_____Times/day

Purpose/ Goal:_____

_____

Comments: Lifting one leg decreases the base of support and changes the center of gravity to challenge balance reactions. Moving the leg around challenges trunk stability while allowing for mobility of the leg .

Hip Lift with Bent Elbows-Spinal Mobility   3:6

Starting Position: Lie on back. Put calves on ball and arms on floor with elbows bent perpendicular with fingers pointing towards ceiling. Press arms into floor and lift buttocks up until body is in a straight line.

Movement/Exercise: Lower to floor by rolling down spine one vertebra at a time. Reverse and curl spine up one vertebra at a time.

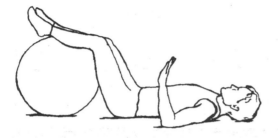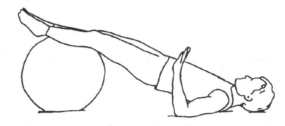

CAUTION: STAY WITHIN PAIN FREE RANGE. DO NOT ARCH BACK.

Breathing: Inhale when lifting, exhale when lowering.

Modification:
1. Place ball closer to buttocks.
2. Lift only as far as comfort and balance allow.

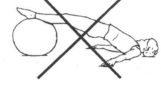

Progression:
1. Place ball farther down legs towards heels.
2. Pick one leg up off ball. Balance, lower leg into ball. Alternate sides.
3. Pick up one leg and write alphabet in the air as big and fast as possible.
4. Add cuff weights at ankles.

Hold____Seconds

Weights_____

Repeat_____ Times

Do_____Times/day

Purpose/ Goal:_____

_____

Comments: Bending elbows changes the center of gravity and lessens the base of support to challenge balance reactions. Lifting one leg further challenges balance reactions while training trunk stability while allowing for mobility of the arms and legs.

Hip Lift with Raised Arms-Spinal Mobility 3:7

Starting Position: Lie on back. Put calves on ball and lift arms off floor at sides or reach for ceiling. Lift buttocks up until body is in a straight line.

Movement/Exercise: Lower to floor by rolling down spine one vertebra at a time. Reverse and curl up spine one vertebra at a time.

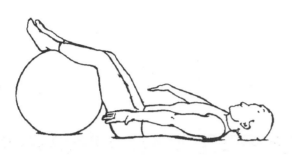 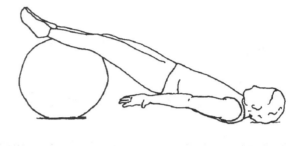

CAUTION: STAY WITHIN PAIN FREE RANGE. DO NOT ARCH BACK.

Breathing: Inhale when lifting, exhale when lowering.

Modification:
1. Place ball closer to buttocks.
2. Lift only as far as comfort and balance allow.

Progression:
1. Place ball farther down legs to heels.
2. Pick one leg up off ball. Balance, lower leg on ball. Alternate sides.
3. Pick up one leg and write alphabet in the air as big and fast as possible.
4. Add cuff weights at ankles.

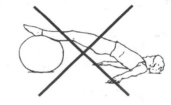

Hold ____Seconds

Weights_____

Repeat_____ Times

Do_____Times/day

Purpose/ Goal:_____

_____

Comments: Lifting arms changes the center of gravity and lessens the base of support to challenge balance reactions. Lifting one leg further challenges balance reactions while training trunk stability and allowing for mobility of the arms and legs.

Date_____   Name_____

Hip Lift-Spinal Stability   3:8

Starting Position: Lie on back. Put calves on ball and hands on floor at side.

Movement/Exercise: Find pain free position of the spine. Press arms into floor and lift trunk as a single unit until body is in a line from ankles to shoulders. Reverse and lower spine to floor as single unit. Distance between hip bone and lowest rib does not change while lifting or lowering body.

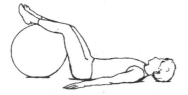 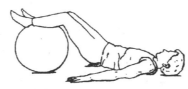 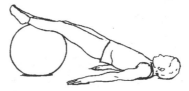

CAUTION: *STAY WITHIN PAIN FREE RANGE. DO NOT ARCH BACK.*

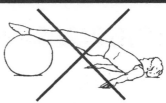

Breathing: Inhale when lifting, exhale when lowering.

Modification:
1. Place ball closer to buttocks.
2. Lift only as far as comfort and balance allow.

Progression:
1. Place ball farther down legs to heels.
2. Pick one leg up off ball. Balance, lower leg on ball. Alternate sides.
3. Pick up one leg and write alphabet in the air as big and fast as possible.
4. Add cuff weights at ankles.

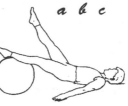

Hold____Seconds

Weights_____

Repeat_____ Times

Do_____Times/day

Purpose/ Goal:_____

_____

Comments: *Lifting one leg decreases the base of support and changes the center of gravity to challenge balance reactions. It also trains trunk stability while allowing for mobility of the legs.*

© 1995 by Joanne Posner-Mayer, PT

Date_____   Name_____

Hip Lift with Bent Elbows-Spinal Stability   3:9

Starting Position: Lie on back. Put calves on ball and arms on floor with elbows bent perpendicular with fingers pointing toward ceiling.

Movement/Exercise: Find pain free position of the spine. Press arms into floor and lift trunk as a single unit until body is in a line from ankles to shoulders. Reverse and lower spine to floor as a single unit.

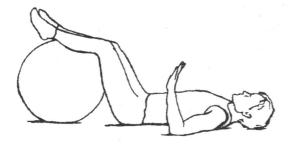 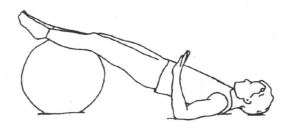

CAUTION: STAY WITHIN PAIN FREE RANGE. DO NOT ARCH BACK.

Breathing: Inhale when lifting, exhale when lowering.

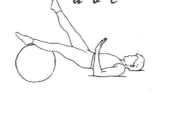

Modification:
1. Place ball closer to buttocks.
2. Lift only as far as comfort and balance allow.

Progression:
1. Place ball farther down legs to heels.
2. Pick one leg up off ball. Balance, lower legs on to ball. Alternate sides.
3. Pick up one leg and write alphabet in the air as big and fast as possible.
4. Add cuff weights at ankles.

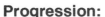

Hold____Seconds

Weights_____

Repeat _____ Times

Do_____Times/day

Purpose/ Goal:_____

_____

Comments: Bending elbows decreases the base of support challenging balance reactions and changing the center of gravity. Lifting one leg further challenges balance reactions while training trunk stability and allowing for mobility of the arms and legs.

© 1995 by Joanne Posner-Mayer, PT

Hip Lift with Raised Arms-Spinal Stability   *3:10*

Starting Position: Lie on back. Put calves on ball and lift arms off floor at sides or reaching for ceiling.

Movement/Exercise: Find pain free position of the spine. Lift trunk as a single unit until body is in a line from ankles to shoulders. Reverse and lower spine as a single unit.

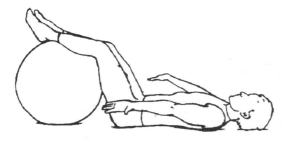

CAUTION: *STAY WITHIN PAIN FREE RANGE. DO NOT ARCH BACK.*

Breathing: Inhale when lifting, exhale when lowering.

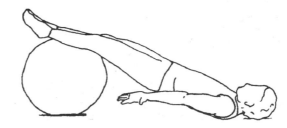

Modification:
1. Place ball closer to buttocks.
2. Lift only as far as comfort and balance allow.

Progression:
1. Place ball farther down legs to heels.
2. Pick one leg up off ball. Balance, lower leg on to ball. Alternate sides.
3. Pick up one leg and write alphabet in the air as big and fast as possible.
4. Add cuff weights at ankles.

Hold ____Seconds

Weights_____

Repeat _____ Times

Do_____Times/day

Purpose/ Goal:_____

_____

Comments: *Lifting arms decreases the base of support challenging balance reactions and changing the center of gravity. Lifting one leg further challenges balance reactions while training trunk stability and allowing for mobility of the arms and legs.*

© 1995 by Joanne Posner-Mayer, PT

Date_____ Name_____

Advanced Hip Lift-Spinal Stability 3:11

Starting Position: Lie on back, and place calves on ball. Find pain free position of spine. Press arms into floor and lift trunk as a single unit until body is in a line from ankles to shoulders. Keeping trunk still, lift one leg slightly off ball.

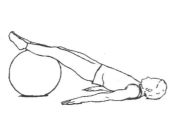 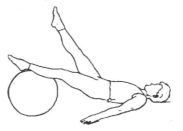

Movement/Exercise: Move leg out to side, allow knee to bend and cross ankle under supporting leg. Straighten knee, returning leg out to side and adduct leg across and above supporting leg. Repeat. Return leg to ball and lower hips to floor.

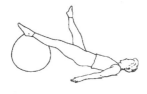 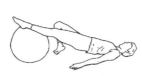 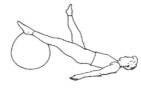 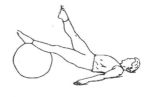

CAUTION: *STAY WITHIN PAIN FREE RANGE. KEEP HIPS PARALLEL TO FLOOR. DO NOT ARCH BACK.*

Breathing: Breathe comfortably. Do not hold breath.

Modification:
1. Lift trunk as far as comfort and balance allow.
2. Reduce range of motion of the leg.

Progression:
1. Place ball farther down legs to heels.
2. To decrease base of support, bend or lift arms off floor.
3. Add cuff weights to ankles.

Hold _____Seconds / Weights_____ / Repeat _____ Times / Do_____Times/day

Purpose/ Goal:_____

_____

Comments: *Moving the leg keeps the center of gravity changing which challenges balance reactions and trunk stability and allows for mobility of the leg. Hip muscle strength can be assessed if hips drop and rise during exercise.*

Chapter 4	Spinal Flexion

Date_____   Name_____

Gentle Abdominals-Sitting   4:1

Starting Position: Sit correctly on the ball in optimal posture.

Movement/Exercise: Turn neck as far as possible to look over one shoulder.
Return to center and repeat to other side.

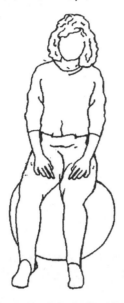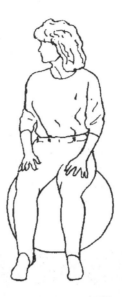

CAUTION: *KEEP FEET PLANTED ON FLOOR.*

Breathing: Inhale on rotation, exhale on return.

Modification: Lightly touch hands to ball or stable object for balance assist.

Progression:
1. Allow ear to lower toward shoulder without turning neck.
2. Close eyes and lower ear toward shoulder and return to center

Hold_____Seconds   /   Repeat_____ Times   /   Do_____Times/day

Purpose/ Goal:_____

_____

Comments: *Turning the head changes the center of gravity and causes abdominal muscles to tighten automatically to maintain balance. The ability to keep the trunk stable while mobilizing the neck is important so the head can move independently of the trunk and gather optimal visual and auditory information.*

Date_____ Name_____

Gentle Abdominals-Rotation   4:2

Starting Position: Lie on back and place calves on top of ball with arms at sides on floor.

Movement/Exercise: Let ball roll as knees rock to one side as far as possible. Tighten abdominals and bring knees back to start. Repeat to other side.

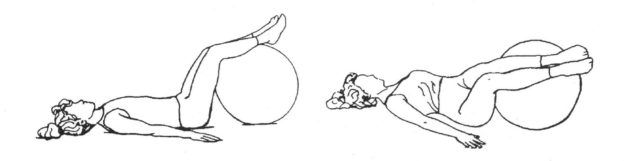

CAUTION: *STAY IN PAIN-FREE RANGE. DO NOT ARCH BACK AT END OF RANGE.*

Breathing: Exhale when lowering, inhale on return.

Modification: Only rock knees through partial range.

Progression:
1. Hold at end range before returning.
2. Lift arms off floor.
3. Simultaneously turn face in the opposite direction of knees.

Hold_____Seconds

Repeat_____ Times

Do_____Times/day

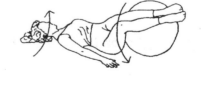

Purpose/ Goal:_____

_____

Comments: *Notice if range is the same on each side. Asymmetries may be due to joint or soft tissue restrictions. The legs get heavier the farther the knees move to the side. The abdominal muscles must activate to resist gravity and keep legs on the ball.*

Date_____   Name_____

Abdominal Curls

Starting Position: Lie on back with knees bent and feet on floor. Place ball on abdomen and hold with both hands.

Movement/Exercise: Use hands to roll ball up to top of knees. Tuck chin toward chest and lift head and shoulders off the floor. Lower to start. Repeat.

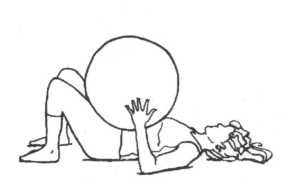 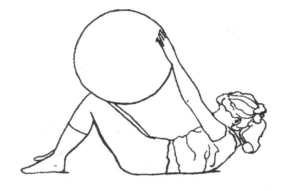

CAUTION: STAY IN PAIN-FREE RANGE. KEEP CHIN A FIST'S DISTANCE FROM CHEST.

Breathing: Exhale while lifting, inhale while lowering.

Modification: Put one hand behind neck to support head or touch fingers of one hand lightly to head but avoid pushing chin to chest.

Progression: Place one hand behind head and one hand on top of ball. Roll ball diagonally across body to outside of opposite knee. Tuck chin toward chest and lift head and shoulder of arm rolling ball.

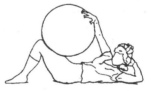

Hold _____ Seconds

Repeat _____ Times

Do_____Times/day

Purpose/ Goal:_____

_____

Comments: *The ball serves as a 1 1/2 to 2lbs weight. Rolling straight targets the rectus abdominis muscle and rolling diagonally targets the oblique abdominal muscles.*

Date_____   Name_____

Half Sit-Up Spinal Mobility   4:4

Starting Position: Sit correctly on ball in optimal posture.

Movement/Exercise: Lean backward and allow ball to roll forward while simultaneously lifting heels and raising arms overhead. Hold.

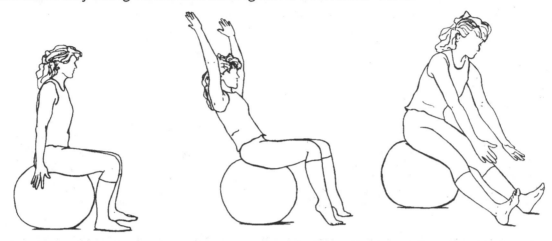

Reverse by leaning forward and straightening knees while lowering arms and rolling the ball backward. Reach fingers toward toes while rocking onto heels and allowing spine to bend. Repeat.

CAUTION: *STAY IN PAIN-FREE RANGE.*

Breathing: Inhale while leaning backward, exhale while moving forward.

Modification: Cross arms over chest or do not fully extend arms overhead.

Progression:
1. Lean farther backward.
2. Add light weights to wrists or hands.

Hold _____Seconds   **Weights_____**

Repeat_____ Times   **Do_____Times/day**

Purpose/ Goal:_____

_____

Comments: *Feel abdominal muscles lengthen (eccentrically contract) while leaning backward and shorten (concentrically contract) while returning to sitting. Back extensor muscles are acting reciprocally while reaching for toes and returning to sit. This exercise may improve the ability to sway forward and backward and recover balance.*

© 1995 by Joanne Posner-Mayer, PT

Date_____ Name_____

Half Sit-Up Spinal Stability   4:5

Starting Position: Sit correctly on ball in optimal posture.

Movement/Exercise: Maintain optimal posture while leaning backward.
Simultaneously lift heels and raise arms overhead letting the ball roll forward. Hold.

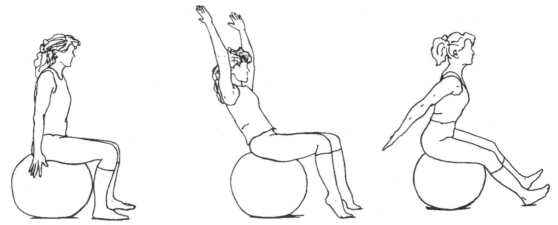

Reverse by leaning forward bending at hips and straightening knees while lowering
arms and rolling ball backward. Maintain optimal posture as straight arms move
behind body with palms facing upward.

CAUTION: *STAY IN PAIN-FREE RANGE. DO NOT ALLOW SPINE TO TWIST
OR BEND.*

Breathing: Inhale while leaning backward, exhale while leaning forward.

Modification: Cross arms over chest or do not fully extend arms.

Progression:
1. Lean farther backward and forward.
2. Add light weights to wrists or hands.

Hold ____Seconds   Weights_____

Repeat_____ Times   Do_____Times/day

Purpose/ Goal:_____

_____

Comments: *Abdominal and back muscles must tighten simultaneously (isometric contraction) to
keep the spine stable while leaning forward and backward. The hip joint acts like a hinge to allow the
spine to sway instead of bending at the low back. The ability to lean forward will depend upon the
flexibility of the hamstring muscles.*

Date_____   Name_____

Half Sit-Up with Obliques-Spinal Stability   4:6

Starting Position: Sit correctly on ball in optimal posture. Maintain this posture while leaning backward. Simultaneously lift heels and raise arms overhead while letting ball roll forward. Hold.

Movement/Exercise: Lower one arm diagonally across body and touch hand to outside of opposite knee. Return arm to overhead position and repeat with other arm.

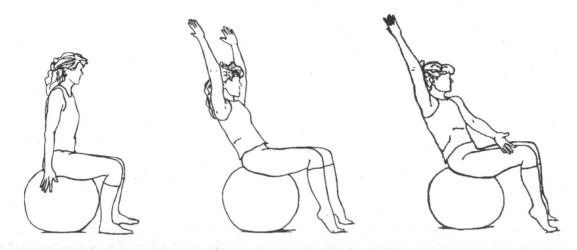

CAUTION: *STAY IN PAIN-FREE RANGE. AVOID TWISTING OR BENDING SPINE.*

Breathing: Inhale while raising arm, exhale while lowering arm.

Modification:
1. Do not fully extend arms.
2. Keep feet flat on floor.

Progression:
1. Lean farther backward.
2. Add light weights to wrist or hands.

Hold_____Seconds   **Weights_____**

Repeats_____ Times   **Do_____Times/day**

Purpose/ Goal:_____

_____

Comments: *This exercise will tighten the abdominal muscles without twisting the spine. When lowering arm, feel oblique muscles tighten more to keep the spine stable on this mobile base of support (the ball). Lifting heels further decreases the base of support which challenges balance.*

Date_____   Name_____

Full Abdominal Curls   4:7

Starting Position: Sit on ball and walk feet forward while leaning backward. Allow ball to roll up spine until ball is under low back. Support head with hands and relax trunk over ball.

Movement/Exercise: Curl up by simultaneously contracting abdominal and buttock muscles. Hold. Slowly curl down to starting position.

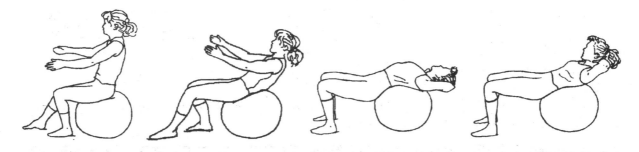

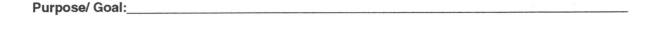

CAUTION: *STAY IN PAIN-FREE RANGE. KEEP CHIN A FIST'S DISTANCE FROM CHEST AND DO NOT PRESS HEAD FORWARD WITH HANDS.*

Breathing: Exhale while lifting, inhale while relaxing.

Modification: Touch fingers lightly to ball or stable object for balance assist.

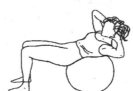

Progression: Curl diagonally across body bringing one shoulder toward opposite hip.

Hold_____Seconds

Repeat_____ Times

Do_____Times/day

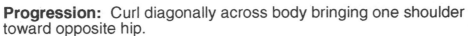

Purpose/ Goal:_____

_____

Comments: Lying over ball challenges balance and allows abdominal muscles to fully lengthen before contracting. Curling straight targets the rectus abdominis while rolling diagonally targets the oblique muscles.

© 1995 by Joanne Posner-Mayer, PT

Dynamic Full Sit-Up   4:8

Starting Position: Sit on ball and place feet forward until knees are straight and feet are flat on floor. Reach arms forward to shoulder level.

Movement/Exercise: Simultaneously bend knees and lean backward (allow ball to roll forward). Keep going until knees are bent 90° and back is in a straight line. Keep arms at sides and squeeze buttocks.

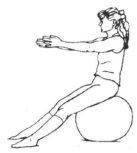 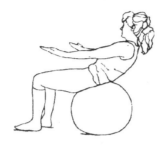 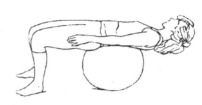

To reverse, push feet into floor, straighten knees and curl trunk up to sitting position allowing ball to roll underneath buttocks.

CAUTION: STAY IN PAIN-FREE RANGE. DO NOT RISE ON TO TOES OR LET HIPS FLEX IN SUPINE POSITION.

Breathing: Inhale while leaning backward, exhale while moving forward.

Modification:
1. Touch ball or stable object while rolling for balance assistance.
2. Only lean back and roll down as far as comfort allows.
3. Place hands behind head to support neck.

Progression:
1. Increase speed of repetitions.
2. Add light weights to wrist or hands.

Hold_____Seconds   Weights_____

Repeat_____ Times   Do_____Times/day

Purpose/ Goal:_____

_____

Comments: *Rolling on the ball while performing an abdominal curl dynamically challenges balance. Adding speed increases the body's momentum mimicking losing and recovering balance. In the end position, the buttock and abdominal muscles should maximally tighten. This trains these muscles to integrate to support and protect the low back.*

© 1995 by Joanne Posner-Mayer, PT

Dynamic Full Sit-Up with Obliques   4:9

Starting Position: Sit correctly on ball in optimal posture and place feet forward until knees are straight and feet are flat on floor. Lift arms in front at shoulder height.

Movement/Exercise: Simultaneously bend knees and lean backward (allow ball to roll forward). While leaning backward, bring one arm out to side and reach other hand across to opposite shoulder. Keep going until knees are bent to 90° and back is in a straight line. Squeeze buttocks.

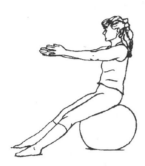 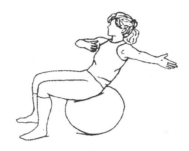 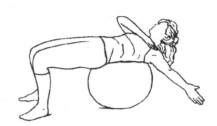

To reverse, push feet into floor, straighten knees and simultaneously curl trunk up to sitting position (allow ball to roll underneath buttocks) while returning arms forward to center. Repeat to other side.

CAUTION: *STAY IN PAIN-FREE RANGE. DO NOT RISE ON TO TOES OR LET HIPS FLEX IN SUPINE POSITION.*

Breathing: Inhale while leaning backward, exhale while moving forward.

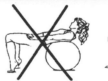

Modification:
1. Move only one arm out to side.
2. Only lean back and roll down as far as comfort allows.

Progression:
1. Increase speed of repetitions.
2. Add weights to arms.

Hold_____Seconds / Weights_____ / Repeat_____ Times / Do_____Times/day

Purpose/ Goal:_____

_____

Comments: *This exercise targets the oblique muscles without twisting the spine. Rolling on the ball while performing an abdominal curl dynamically challenges balance. Adding speed increases the body's momentum mimicking losing and recovering balance. In the end position, the buttock and abdominal muscles should maximally tighten. This trains these muscles to integrate to support and protect the low back.*

Chapter 5 — Core Control

Date_____   Name_____

Ball Hug   5:1

Starting Position: Sit on edge of chair or bench with ball resting in lap against chest. Place arms around widest part of ball.

Movement/Exercise: Lift ball off lap until hands are even with shoulders and hug ball to chest. Hold. Lower to starting position. Repeat.

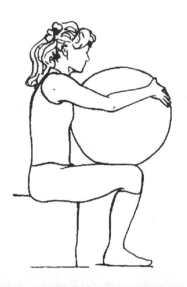 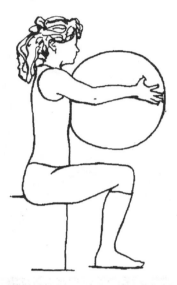

CAUTION: *KEEP SHOULDERS DOWN WHILE LIFTING AND HUGGING BALL WITH HANDS.*

Breathing: Inhale while lifting and squeezing, exhale while lowering.

Modification: Extend knees and squeeze ball into stomach.

Hold_____Seconds

Repeat_____ Times

Do_____Times/day

Purpose/ Goal:_____

_____

Comments: *Feel spine straighten as ball is lifted and squeezed. Besides activating spinal stabilizers, the scapular muscles between shoulder blades and shoulder joint muscles are required to tighten.*

Date_____   Name_____

Gentle Trunk Isometric-Supine   5:2

Starting Position: Place ball close to wall and lie down next to it with knees bent and feet on floor. Adjust ball so that it is lightly pressed between the wall and knees. If no wall is available, use arm to hold ball at side.

Movement/Exercise: Press knees against ball as hard as is comfortable. Hold. Relax and repeat. Switch sides.

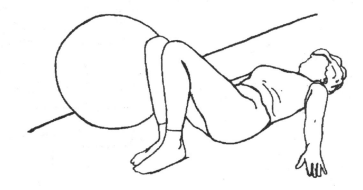

CAUTION: *STAY IN PAIN-FREE RANGE AND DO NOT ARCH BACK.*

Breathing: Inhale while pressing, exhale while relaxing.

Modification: Sit in a chair and press knees against ball holding it still with hand or wall.

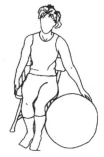

Progression: Tie resistive band around knees and open knees apart pressing one knee into ball and other out to side.

Hold____Seconds

Repeat_____ Times

Do_____Times/day

Purpose/ Goal:_____

_____

Comments: *Feel oblique abdominal muscles tighten along with spinal stabilizers in an isometric contraction. This exercise targets spinal rotator muscles without rotating spine.*

Date_____   Name_____

Push-Up

Starting Position: Kneel behind ball, lie trunk over ball and place hands on floor under shoulders. Walk out on hands letting the ball roll down body and legs as far as strength/balance allows. Keeping spine in optimal posture.

Movement/Exercise: Lower body by bending elbows while balancing on the ball. Push body up by straightening elbows. Repeat. Keep spine still by tightening abdominal and buttock muscles.

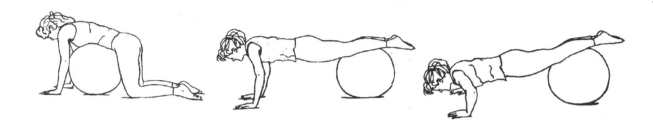

CAUTION: *DO NOT LET LOWER BACK SAG OR BEND AT HIPS. KEEP FACE PARALLEL TO THE FLOOR. TRY TO PERFORM EXERCISE ON PADDED SURFACE SUCH AS CARPET, MATS OR BOTH. AVOID LOCKING ELBOWS WHEN RESTING.*

Breathing: Inhale while lowering, exhale while raising. Do not hold breath.

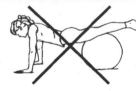

Modification:
1. Have someone assist by lightly touching legs for balance.
2. Walk out on fisted hands if stress is too great on wrists.

Progression:
1. Increase speed.
2. Lift up one leg.

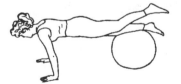

Hold____Seconds / Repeat_____ Times / Do_____Times/day

Purpose/ Goal:_____

_____

Comments: *This exercise is a weight bearing kinetic chain for the arms and shoulders. Notice that the closer the ball is to the feet the more strenuous this exercise becomes on arms and trunk as body maintains balance while lowering and raising up.*

Date_____ Name_____

Advanced Push-Up   *5:4*

Starting Position: Assume standard push-up position on toes and place hands on top of ball in line with shoulders. Maintain optimal posture and balance.

Movement/Exercise: Controlling ball, bend arms and lower trunk as far as possible without losing balance. Straighten arms and return to starting position. Repeat.

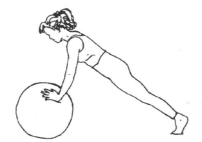 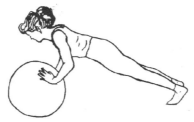 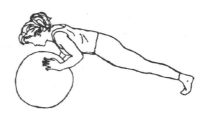

CAUTION: *STAY WITHIN PAIN-FREE RANGE. KEEP NECK IN OPTIMAL POSITION.*

Breathing: Inhale while lowering, exhale while pressing up.

Modification: Perform with bent knees on floor.

Progression: Increase speed of repetitions.

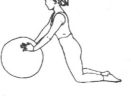 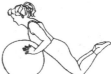

Hold ____Seconds

Repeat_____ Times

Do_____Times/day

Purpose/ Goal:_____

_____

Comments: *Feel the tightening of spinal extensor, flexor and shoulder girdle muscles. The ball provides an unstable base of support which significantly increases the difficulty of a push up.*

© 1995 by Joanne Posner-Mayer, PT

Date_____   Name_____

Prone Walk-Out   5:5

Starting Position: Kneel behind ball. Lie trunk over ball and place hands on floor under shoulders.

Movement/Exercise: Walk out on hands letting the ball roll down body. Walk out as far as strength/balance allows and return to starting position. Keep spine in optimal posture by tightening abdominals and buttocks.

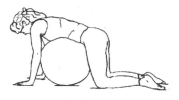 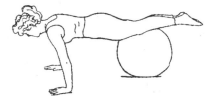 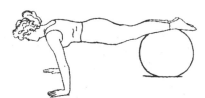

CAUTION: *DO NOT LET LOWER BACK SAG OR BEND AT HIPS. KEEP FACE PARALLEL TO THE FLOOR. TRY TO PERFORM EXERCISE ON PADDED SURFACE SUCH AS CARPET, MATS OR BOTH.*

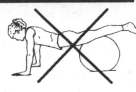

Breathing: Breathe comfortably. Do not hold breath.

Modification:
1. Have someone assist by lightly touching legs for balance.
2. Walk out on fisted hands if stress is too great on wrists.

Progression:
1. Gently rock forward and backward.
2. When at end position, balance and lift up one leg.
3. Write the alphabet with foot of lifted leg.

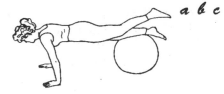

Hold_____Seconds / Repeat_____ Times / Do_____Times/day

Purpose/ Goal:_____

_____

Comments: This exercise is a weight bearing kinetic chain for the arms and shoulders. Notice that the farther one walks out on the ball the exercise becomes more strenuous on the upper body and trunk as they adjust to keep the body balanced as the lever arm increases.

Total Body Flexion   5:6

Starting Position: Assume prone walkout position (exercise 5:5). Keep spine in optimal posture and allow ball to roll down legs until knee caps are just on top of ball.

Movement/Exercise: Simultaneously, pull in stomach, lift hips and bend knees. Roll ball forward underneath trunk until shins rest on ball. Relax trunk in full flexion for a few moments before straightening knees and hips to return to start. Repeat.

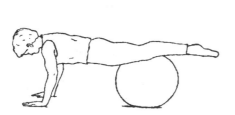 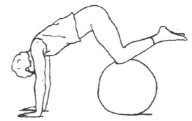 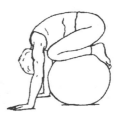

CAUTION: *AFTER A FEW REPETITIONS, BALL POSITION MAY NEED TO BE ADJUSTED AS IT MAY SLIDE ON CLOTHES. TRY TO PERFORM EXERCISE ON PADDED SURFACE SUCH AS CARPET, MATS OR BOTH.*

Breathing: Inhale as body flexes, exhale as body extends.

Modification:
1. Have someone assist by lightly holding ankles for balance.
2. Perform through partial range only if flexion restriction or discomfort exist.
3. Walk out on fisted hands if stress is too great on wrists.

Progression:
1. Increase speed and do not pause on top of ball before reversing.
2. Have an assistant add resistance to movement by holding ankles and walking forward and backward resisting movement.

Hold _____Seconds   **Weights_____**

Repeat _____ Times   **Do_____Times/day**

Purpose/ Goal:_____

_____

Comments: This exercise is a weight bearing kinetic chain for the arms and shoulders. Notice how strenuous this exercise is on the upper body as it adjusts to keep the body balanced and to coordinate this exercise while the base of support, lever arm and center of gravity continually change. Increasing speed increases momentum.

© 1995 by Joanne Posner-Mayer, PT

Date_____   Name_____

Total Body Extension   5:7

Starting Position: Assume prone walkout position (exercise 5:5). Keep spine in optimal posture and allow ball to roll down legs until knee caps are just on top of ball.

Movement/Exercise: Press hands into floor and lift feet as body pushes back (do not move hands). Allow ball to roll up body to support pelvis. Extend spine as far as strength and comfort allow. Lower head between arms. Reverse motion by tightening abdominal muscles to initiate. Return to starting position (do not let lower back sag).

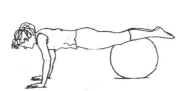 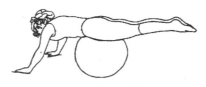 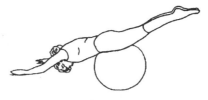

CAUTION: *AVOID LIFTING FEET TOO HIGH AS IT WILL RESULT IN OVER ARCHING THE LOWER BACK. STAY IN PAIN FREE RANGE.*

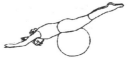

Breathing: Inhale on roll back, exhale on roll forward.

Modification:
1. Have someone assist by lightly holding ankles for balance.
2. Perform through partial range only if restriction exists.
3. Only walk out as far as comfort allows.

Progression:
1. Combine total body flexion and extension into a fluid movement sequence (inhaling on flexion, exhaling on extension).
2. Have an assistant add resistance to movement by holding ankles and walking forward and backward during movement.

Hold ____Seconds

Repeat_____ Times / Do_____Times/day

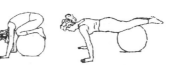

Purpose/ Goal:_____

_____

Comments: *This exercise is a weight bearing kinetic chain for the arms and shoulders. Notice how strenuous this exercise is on the upper body and abdomen as it adjusts to keep body balanced and to coordinate this exercise while the base of support, lever arm and center of gravity continually change.*

Prone Skier   5:8

Starting Position: Assume Prone Walk-Out position (exercise 5:5). Keep spine in optimal posture until knees are just past the top of the ball.

Movement/Exercise: Keep shoulders parallel to the floor as hips are lifted and turned. Let ball roll as knees are pulled under trunk on a diagonal aimed toward underarm. To reverse, straighten knees and return to starting position keeping hips lifted. Repeat to other side.

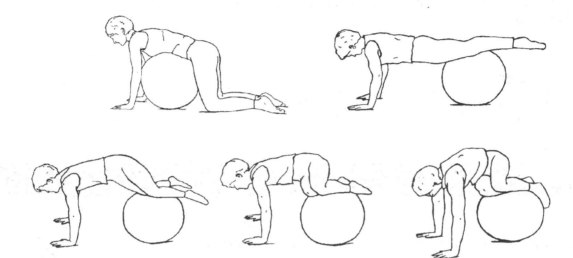

CAUTION: *MUST BE ABLE TO PERFORM TOTAL BODY FLEXION (SEE PAGE 114) BEFORE ATTEMPTING THIS EXERCISE. EXERCISE CANNOT BE PERFORMED WITH BALL UNDER THIGHS. DO NOT LET BACK SAG ON RETURN TO STARTING POSITION.*

Breathing: Inhale as knees are pulled up, exhale as knees are extended.

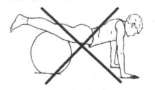

Modification: Only pull knees up as far as is comfortable for back and/or knees.

Progression:
1. Increase speed.
2. Have an assistant hold and walk along giving resistance to movement.

Beats/min_____ / Repeat_____ Times / Do_____Times/day

Purpose/ Goal:_____

Comments: *This exercise is a weight bearing and strengthening exercise for the shoulder girdle. Notice how strenuous this exercise is on the abdominals and shoulder girdle as they maintain balance while absorbing momentum. If it is easier to one side, it can be due to restricted spinal rotation or shoulder girdle weakness.*

© 1995 by Joanne Posner-Mayer, PT

Date_____   Name_____

Hip Twister   5:9

Starting Position: Assume Prone Walk-Out position (exercise 5:5) until ball is under knees.

Movement/Exercise: Keeping shoulders parallel to floor, turn pelvis perpendicular to floor and lift upper leg. Slowly reverse to return to starting position and repeat to other side.

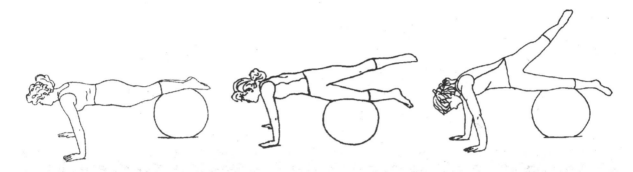

CAUTION: KEEP LEGS IN STRAIGHT LINE WITH TORSO. DO NOT BEND AT HIPS OR LET UPPER LEG MOVE FORWARD OR BACKWARD.

Breathing: Inhale while twisting, exhale while returning.

Modification:
1. Roll ball to hips.
2. Keep legs together.
3. Do not turn fully.
4. Have someone give balance assist by holding ankles.

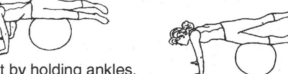

Progression: Roll ball past knees and follow movement instructions.

Beats/min_____

Repeat_____ Times

Do_____Times/day

Purpose/ Goal:_____

_____

Comments: This exercise is a weight bearing and strengthening exercise for the shoulder girdle. Notice how strenuous this exercise is on the abdominals and shoulder girdle as they maintain balance while absorbing momentum. If it is easier to one side, it can be due to restricted spinal rotation or shoulder girdle weakness.

Log Roll   5:10

Starting Position: Assume Prone Walk-Out position (exercise 5:5) until knees are resting on the ball.

Movement/Exercise: Let ball roll and sway hips and legs as far as possible to one side without losing balance. Repeat to other side.

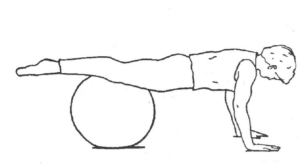 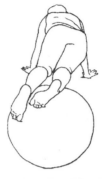

CAUTION: *KEEP SPINE IN OPTIMAL ALIGNMENT! DO NOT ARCH NECK OR BACK.*

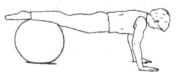

Breathing: Do not hold breath. Breathe comfortably.

Modification:
1. Only walk out until thighs are resting on ball.
2. Have someone assist balance by holding ankles.

Progression:
1. Increase speed of sway and recovery.
2. Walk out until ankles rest on ball.
3. Have an assistant add resistance on sway and recovery.

Beats/min_____

Repeat_____ Times

Do_____Times/day

Purpose/ Goal:_____

_____

Comments: *This is a non-weight bearing exercise for the legs that mimics the lateral sway and recovery pattern of the trunk while standing. Notice how strenuous this exercise is on the abdominals and shoulders as they maintain balance while absorbing momentum. It is also a weight bearing kinetic chain exercise for the arms and shoulder girdle.*

Date_____ Name_____

Table Top Supine   5:11

Starting Position: Sit on ball and raise arms in front of body to shoulder height.

Movement/Exercise: Simultaneously walk feet out and lean backward allowing ball to roll up back until ball is under head and neck (as if on a pillow). Lift straight arms overhead so they are in a straight line with body when fully supine. Hold. Reverse by walking feet backward and curl trunk up to sitting position and relax. Repeat.

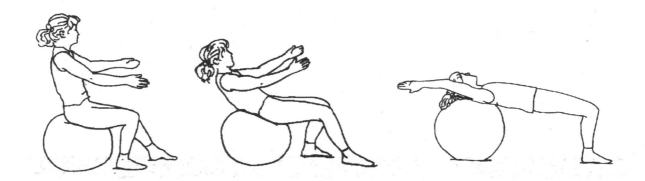

CAUTION: *DO NOT OVEREXTEND SPINE OR SAG AT HIPS.*

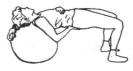

Breathing: Do not hold breath. Breathe comfortably.

Modification:
1. Clasp hands behind head for support. Walk out until ball is underneath shoulder blades.
2. Touch hands to ball and then to floor for balance assist.

Progression:
1. Hold arms out to side.
2. Keeping both feet on the floor, shift weight from one foot to the other.

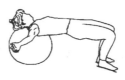

Repeat_____ Times   Do_____Times/day

Purpose/ Goal:_____

_____

Comments: *This exercise is gentle to the spine yet recruits spinal stabilizers to maintain balance. It is also a weight bearing kinetic chain exercise for the legs.*

Advanced Table-Top Supine   5:12

Starting Position: Assume Supine Table-Top position (exercise 5:11).

Movement/Exercise: Pick up one foot and straighten knee until leg is parallel with floor. Hold. Return and switch legs.

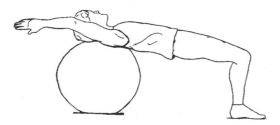
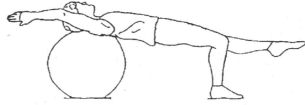

CAUTION: *DO NOT OVEREXTEND SPINE OR SAG AT HIPS.*

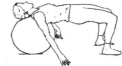

Breathing: Do not hold breath. Breathe comfortably.

Modification:
1. Clasp hands behind head for support. Walk out until ball is underneath shoulder blades.
2. Touch hands to ball and then to floor for balance assistance.
3. Have assistant hold wrists overhead for balance assistance.

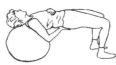

Progression:
1. Hold arms out to side.
2. Write alphabet with non-weight bearing foot. Increase speed and size to add more difficulty.

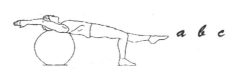

Repeat_____ Times   Do_____Times/day

Purpose/ Goal:_____

_____

Comments: *This exercise is gentle to the spine yet recruits spinal stabilizers to maintain balance. It is a weight bearing kinetic chain exercise for the legs. Writing the alphabet adds random perturbations to challenge balance and proprioception while adding momentum and inertia. This exercise mimics standing on one leg and recovering balance when it is unexpectedly perturbed.*

Chapter 6 — Lower Extremity

Date_____   Name_____

Hip Flexor Stretch   6:1

Starting Position: Kneel behind ball with hands on ball. Bring one foot as far forward beside ball as comfort allows. Form an angle of at least 90° at hip and knee.

Movement/Exercise: Place elbows on ball under shoulders and allow ball to roll forward as far as comfort allows. Allow ribs to rest on ball. Return, rest and repeat. Change sides. Feel stretch in hip flexor as the ball rolls forward.

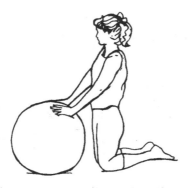 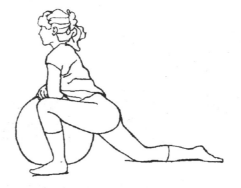

CAUTION: *KEEP FRONT KNEE IN LINE WITH TOES. DO NOT ALLOW KNEE TO PASS FARTHER FORWARD THAN TOES. STAY IN PAIN FREE RANGE.*

Breathing: Do not hold breath. Breathe comfortably.

Modification: Allow trunk to rest fully on the ball. Let hands touch floor.

Progression: Dig toes of back leg into floor and straighten knee. Reach backward with heel to stretch calf muscles.

Hold____Seconds

Repeat_____ Times

Do_____Times/day

Purpose/ Goal:_____

_____

Comments: *The ball supports the weight of the body and stabilizes the spine as the hip flexor muscle is gently stretched with the help of gravity.*

Date_____ Name_____

Hip Extensor Stretch-Supine   6:2

Starting Position: Lie on floor and, keeping knees straight, place heels on ball one at a time . Cross right ankle over left knee letting it relax out to side.

Movement/Exercise: Bend the left knee toward chest and roll ball toward buttocks. Hold. Return, rest and repeat. Switch legs.

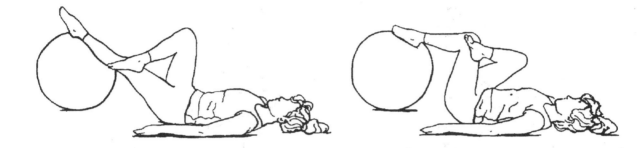

CAUTION: *KEEP HIPS AND BACK ON FLOOR. STAY IN PAIN-FREE RANGE.*

Breathing: Do not hold breath. Breathe comfortably.

Hold_____Seconds

Repeat_____ Times

Do_____Times/day

Purpose/ Goal:_____

_____

Comments: *The ball allows an easily controlled gravity assisted stretch for the hip extensor and internal rotator muscles.*

© 1995 by Joanne Posner-Mayer, PT

Date_____   **Name**_____

Table Top Stretch 6:3

Starting Position: Assume Table Top Supine position (exercise 5:11). Keep hips in line with knees and shoulders by tightening buttocks. Touch hands to floor.

Movement/Exercise: Slide one foot toward ball allowing heel to lift while dropping knee toward floor. Hold. Return, rest and repeat. Switch sides.

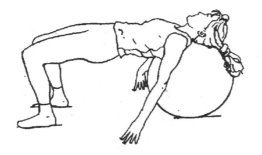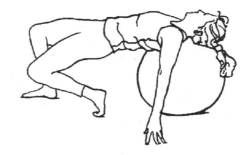

CAUTION: *KEEP SPINE IN OPTIMAL POSTURE. DO NOT ALLOW HIPS TO DROP.*

Breathing: Do not hold breath. Breathe comfortably.

Modification: Touch hands to ball while walking out and then allow hands to touch floor for balance assist while stretching.

Hold_____**Seconds**

Repeat_____ **Times**

Do_____**Times/day**

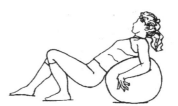

Purpose/ Goal:_____

_____

Comments: *Feel stretch in front of thigh muscle (quadriceps). The ball allows a gravity assisted stretch with precise control of amount of stretch.*

© 1995 by Joanne Posner-Mayer, PT

Date_____   **Name**_____

Hamstring Stretch-Supine   6:4

Starting Position: Lie on back with calves on ball.

Movement/Exercise: Straighten one knee and lift leg off ball as far as comfort allows. Hold. Return, rest and repeat. Switch sides.

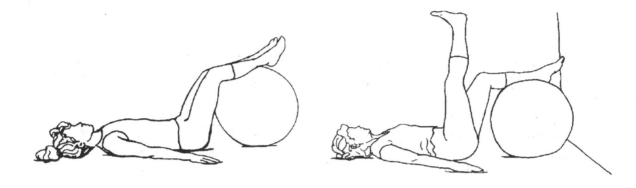

CAUTION: KEEP BUTTOCKS AND LOW BACK ON FLOOR.

Breathing: Do not hold breath. Breathe comfortably.

Modification: Use resistive band to lift leg for strength assist.

Progression: Flex ankle to increase stretch.

Hold_____Seconds

Repeat_____ Times

Do_____Times/day

Purpose/ Goal:_____

_____

Comments: This position allows comfortable support of the spine and other leg as the hips are stabilized and the hamstring muscles experience a targeted yet easily controlled gravity assisted stretch activated by the qaudriceps muscle.

Date_____   Name_____

Bent Knee and Hip Lift-Spinal Mobility   6:5

Starting Position: With knees bent, lie on back and, one at a time, put soles of feet on ball.

Movement/Exercise: Press feet into ball. Tuck hips under and curl spine up one vertebra at a time until knees, hips and shoulders are in a straight line. Slowly return to floor rolling down one vertebra at a time. Repeat.

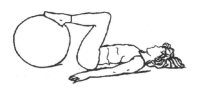 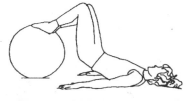 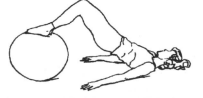

CAUTION: *IF THERE IS ANY LEG CRAMPING, SLOWLY REVERSE AND RELAX. DO NOT ARCH BACK. STAY IN PAIN FREE RANGE.*

Breathing: Do not hold breath. Breathe comfortably.

Modification: Only lift hips to partial range.

Progression:
1. Decrease arm support on floor.
     a. Bend elbows.
     b. Lift arms off floor.

Hold ____Seconds

Repeat_____ Times

Do_____Times/day

Purpose/ Goal:_____

_____

Comments: *Not only does this exercise strengthen the knee flexors and hip extensors, it also challenges balance and trunk control while allowing movement between vertebrae.*

Date_____ Name_____

Bent Knee and Hip Lift-Spinal Stability 6:6

Starting Position: With knees bent, lie on back and, one at a time, put soles of feet on ball.

Movement/Exercise: Maintaining optimal posture, press feet into ball and lift hips and lower back as a unit until knees, hips and shoulders are in a straight line. Slowly reverse to return to start. Repeat.

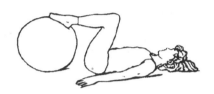 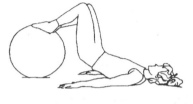 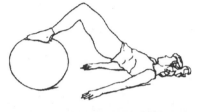

CAUTION: *IF THERE IS ANY LEG CRAMPING, SLOWLY REVERSE AND RELAX. DO NOT ARCH BACK. STAY IN PAIN FREE RANGE.*

Breathing: Do not hold breath. Breathe comfortably.

Modification: Only lift hips to partial range.

Progression:
1. Decrease arm support on floor.
   a. Bend elbows.
   b. Lift arms off floor.

Beats/min_____

Repeat_____ Times

Do_____Times/day

Purpose/ Goal:_____

_____

Comments: *Not only does this exercise strengthen the knee flexors and hip extensors, it also challenges balance and trunk control while not allowing movement of vertebrae.*

Date_____ Name_____

Straight Leg Ball Lift 6:7

Starting Position: Lie on back with knees bent. Prop head and shoulders up on elbows. Grasp ball between ankles.

Movement/Exercise: Tighten abdominal muscles and squeeze ball. Keeping knees straight, lift ball as high as comfort allows. Slowly lower ball to floor and repeat.

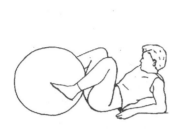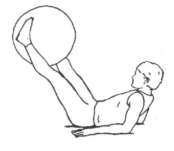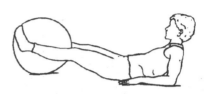

CAUTION: STAY WITHIN PAIN FREE RANGE. DO NOT ALLOW BACK TO ARCH.

Breathing: Do not hold breath. Breathe comfortably.

Modification: Only lift ball to partial range. Hands can be placed under buttocks to increase low back stability.

Progression: Lie with head and shoulders on floor. This adds difficulty to maintain spinal stability in optimal posture.

Hold_____Seconds

Repeat_____ Times

Do_____Times/day

Purpose/ Goal:_____

_____

Comments: This exercise also activates hip adductor muscles.

Date_____ **Name**_____

Frog Legs Supine 6:8

Starting Position: Lie on back with knees bent. Prop head and shoulders up on elbows. Grasp ball between ankles and lift off floor. Bring knees towards chest.

Movement/Exercise: Tighten abdominal muscles and squeeze ball. Straighten hips and knees so that ball moves in a diagonal line. Bend hips and knees back toward chest to return. Repeat . Return to start. Rest.

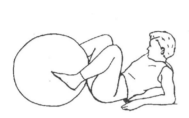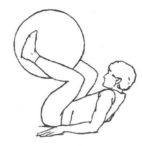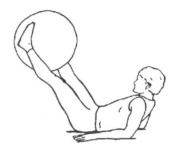

CAUTION: *STAY WITHIN PAIN-FREE RANGE. DIFFICULTY INCREASES AS LEGS ARE STRAIGHTENED. DO NOT ALLOW BACK TO ARCH.*

Breathing: Exhale as legs extend, inhale as legs bend.

Modification: Straighten knees and hips only as far as comfortable.

Progression: Lie with head and shoulders on floor. This adds difficulty to maintain spinal stability in optimal posture.

Hold_____Seconds

Repeat_____ Times

Do_____Times/day

Purpose/ Goal:_____

_____

Comments: *This exercise also activates hip adductor muscles.*

Date_____   Name_____

Leg Press-Supine   6:9

Starting Position: Lie on back with knees bent. Grasp ball between ankles and raise ball off floor.

Movement/Exercise: Tighten abdominal muscles and squeeze ball. Straighten knees and lift ball toward ceiling. Hold. Bend knees toward chest. Repeat. Return to start. Rest.

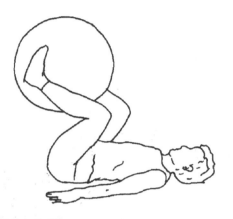 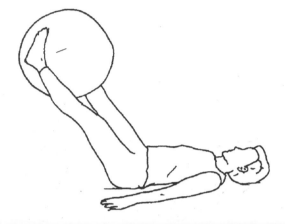

CAUTION: STAY WITHIN PAIN-FREE RANGE. DO NOT ALLOW BACK TO ARCH.

Breathing: Exhale as legs straighten, inhale on return.

Modification: Straighten knees only as far as comfort allows.

Progression: To increase abdominal muscle participation, prop on elbows to lift head and shoulders off floor. Maintain proper neck alignment.

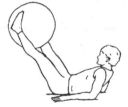

Hold_____Seconds

Repeat_____ Times

Do_____Times/day

Purpose/ Goal:_____

_____

Comments: This exercise also activates hip adductor and abdominal muscles .

Date_____   Name_____

Leg Rotation with Ball   6:10

Starting Position: Lie on back. Prop head and shoulders up on elbows. Grasp ball between knees.

Movement/Exercise: Tighten abdominal muscles and squeeze ball between calves. Lift ball and straighten knees while squeezing ball. Rotate legs by crossing one under the ball and one on top of the ball.

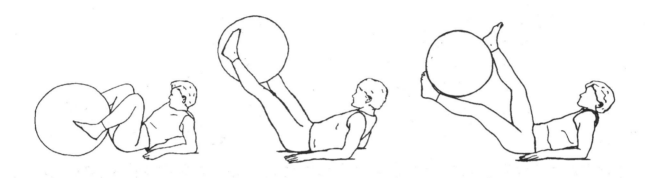

CAUTION: STAY WITHIN PAIN-FREE RANGE. DO NOT ALLOW BACK TO ARCH.

Breathing: Exhale as legs cross, inhale as legs spread apart. Breathe comfortably.

Modification: Bend knees slightly.

Progression: Lie with head and shoulders on floor. This adds difficulty to maintain the low back in optimal posture.

Hold_____Seconds

Repeat_____ Times

Do_____Times/day

Purpose/ Goal:_____

_____

Comments: *This exercise also activates hip adductor and abductor muscles.*

© 1995 by Joanne Posner-Mayer, PT

Date_____   Name_____

Side Lying Ball Lift 6:11

Starting Position: Lie on side in a straight line with knees straight. Place one arm under head and other arm in front for balance. Grasp ball between calves. Stabilize spine and squeeze ball.

Movement/Exercise: Pressing ball up with lower leg, lift both legs off floor as high as comfort allows. Slowly lower ball to floor and repeat.

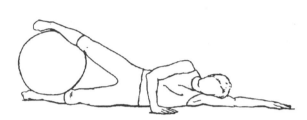 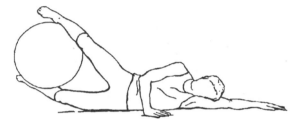

CAUTION: *STAY WITHIN PAIN-FREE RANGE. KEEP SPINE AND LEGS IN A STRAIGHT LINE.*

Breathing: Exhale while lifting, inhale while lowering.

Modification: Bend knees slightly.

Hold_____Seconds

Repeat_____ Times

Do_____Times/day

Purpose/ Goal:_____

_____

Comments: *This exercise also activates hip adductor and abductor muscles as well as challenging balance and trunk stability.*

Side Stretch and Leg Lift   *6:12*

Starting Position: Lie over ball sideways as in end of Side Stretch (exercise 2:10).

Movement/Exercise: Simultaneously lift leg up and reach fingers for toes while lifting trunk. Hold. Slowly reverse to return. Repeat. Switch sides.

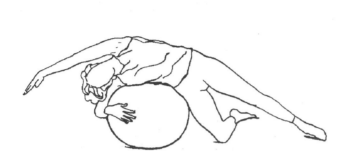 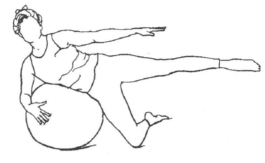

CAUTION: *STAY WITHIN PAIN-FREE RANGE. KEEP LEG IN STRAIGHT LINE WITH SPINE AND KNEE FACING FORWARD.*

Breathing: Exhale while lifting, inhale while returning.

Modification: Only lift as far as comfortable.

Progression:
1. Add cuff weights.
2. Put both hands behind head.

Beats/min_____

Weights_____

Repeat_____ Times

Do_____Times/day

Purpose/ Goal:_____

_____

Comments: *This exercise allows the lateral trunk and hip muscles to start in a fully elongated position and contract to a fully shortened position.*

Date_____ Name_____

Push and Pull Sitting 6:13

Starting Position: Sit on ball in optimal posture. Pick up uninjured leg.

Movement/Exercise: Push support foot into floor and let ball roll forward as support knee is bent and straightened.

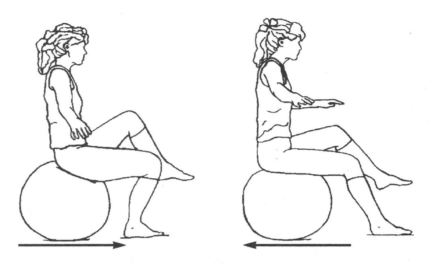

CAUTION: *STAY WITHIN PAIN-FREE RANGE. KEEP SUPPORT KNEE IN LINE WITH FOOT. DO NOT BEND KNEE MORE THAN 90° UNLESS DIRECTED BY THERAPIST.*

Breathing: Do not hold breath. Breathe comfortably.

Modification: Touch hands to ball or stable object for balance assistance.

Progression:
1. Move in diagonals and/or circles.
2. Try to draw alphabet with buttocks.
3. Add speed.

Hold____Seconds

Repeat_____ Times

Do_____Times/day

Purpose/ Goal:_____

_____

Comments: *This is a partial weight bearing exercise which challenges balance and proprioception while increasing strength in the quadriceps muscle. Faster movement adds momentum and velocity that the hips and knees have to control in order to stop and reverse directions.*

Alphabet Sitting 6:14

Starting Position: Sit on ball in optimal posture. Raise arms out to sides. Pick up uninjured leg.

Movement/Exercise: Push into floor with support leg and write *cursive* alphabet with foot of unweighted leg.

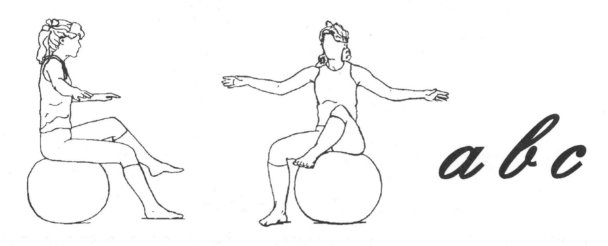

CAUTION: *STAY WITHIN PAIN-FREE RANGE. KEEP SUPPORT KNEE IN LINE WITH TOES. DO NOT BEND MORE THAN 90° UNLESS DIRECTED BY THERAPIST.*

Breathing: Do not hold breath. Breathe comfortably.

Modification: Touch hands to ball or stable object for balance assistance.

Progression:
1. Write alphabet larger and/or faster.
2. Add cuff weight to ankle.

Hold ____Seconds

Repeat_____ Times

Do_____Times/day

Purpose/ Goal:_____

_____

Comments: *This is a partial weight bearing exercise which challenges balance, proprioception and knee stability. Feel how weight bearing leg has to coactivate muscle groups as momentum and size of letters increase.*

Date_____   Name_____

Alphabet-Standing   6:15

Starting Position: Stand in optimal posture. Pick up uninjured leg and place on ball.

Movement/Exercise: Write alphabet with uninjured leg using the ball as a dynamic base of support.

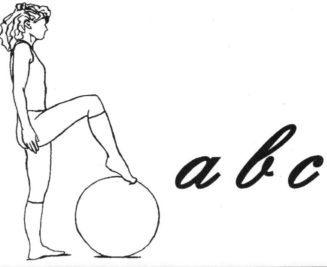

CAUTION: STAY WITHIN PAIN-FREE RANGE. KEEP SUPPORT KNEE IN LINE WITH TOES.

Breathing: Do not hold breath. Breathe comfortably.

Modification: Touch hands to wall or stable object for balance assistance.

Progression: Write alphabet larger and/or faster.

Beats/min_____

Repeat _____ Times

Do_____Times/day

Purpose/ Goal:_____

_____

Comments: *This is a full weight bearing exercise which challenges balance and proprioception while increasing stability in the leg. Notice how trunk and weight bearing leg have to increasingly coactivate muscles as momentum increases.*

Chapter 7 — Upper Extremity

Shoulder Flexion   7:1

Starting Position: Kneel behind ball with hands on top of ball. Walk hands out and let ball roll as body leans forward and trunk curls down.

Movement/Exercise: Go out as far as comfort allows. Keep head between arms and eyes focused on floor.

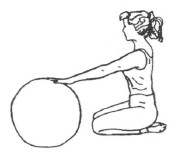

CAUTION: *STAY WITHIN PAIN FREE RANGE.*

Breathing: Exhale while rolling forward, inhale while returning.

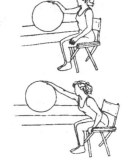

Modification:
1. If there is discomfort in shoulders, bend elbows out to side.
2. If unable to sit on heels, kneel or sit in chair with ball in front on a bed or table.
3. Where weakness exists, roll ball as far as possible orcomfortable then tighten shoulder flexor muscles as if to lift hand off ball.

Progression: At end range, tighten shoulder flexors and lift hand slightly off ball.

Hold_____Seconds   /   Repeat_____ Times   /   Do_____Times/day

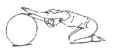

Purpose/ Goal:_____

_____

Comments: The ball allows precise control of this gravity-assisted stretch and allows the stretch to be comfortably maintained. Attempting to lift hand off the ball adds a strengthening exercise.

Date_____   Name_____

Shoulder Extension 7:2

Starting Position: Kneel behind ball with hand on top of ball.

Movement/Exercise: Roll ball backward as far as possible with hand. Hold. Return and relax.

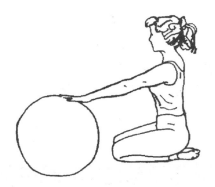 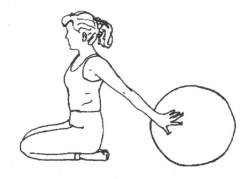

CAUTION: STAY WITHIN PAIN FREE RANGE.

Breathing: Inhale while rolling out, exhale while returning.

Modification:
1. If unable to kneel, sit in chair with ball to side on bed.
2. Where weakness exists, roll ball as far as is possible/comfortable and tighten shoulder extensor muscles.

 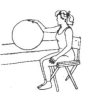

Progression:
1. At end range, roll ball as far as is possible and tighten shoulder extensor muscles for an end range isometric exercise.
2. Lean trunk backward slightly for a gravity assisted stretch.

Hold _____Seconds

Repeat_____ Times

Do_____Times/day

Purpose/ Goal:_____

_____

Comments: *The ball allows precise control of this stretch and allows the stretch to be comfortably maintained. This can also be used to assist scapular adductor muscles. Tightening arm muscles adds a strengthening element to the exercise.*

Date_____   Name_____

Shoulder Abduction   7:3

Starting Position: Kneel next to ball and place hand on top of ball.

Movement/Exercise: Roll ball sideways away from body so that elbow is straight. Continue rolling ball while allowing trunk to bend sideways until arm is in full abduction. Let head rest on abducted arm. Hold. Slowly return to start.

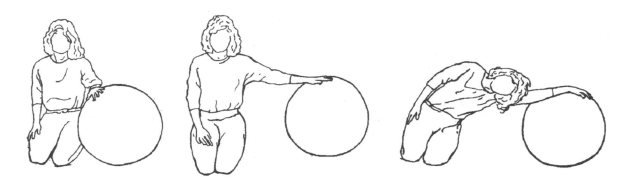

CAUTION: *STAY IN PAIN FREE RANGE.*

Breathing: Do not hold breath. Breathe comfortably.

Modification:
1. Put free hand on floor in front for support and balance assist.
2. Use free hand to support/guide arm on ball.
3. Sit on sofa or bed with ball on same surface.
4. Where weakness exists, roll ball as far as is possible/comfortable and tighten shoulder abductor muscles as if to lift arm off ball.

Progression:
1. With arm extended, roll ball forward and backward to combine internal and external rotation with abduction.
2. At end range, attempt to lift arm off ball for an end range isometric exercise.

Hold____Seconds   /   Repeat_____ Times   /   Do_____Times/day

Purpose/ Goal:_____

_____

Comments: *The ball allows precise control of this gravity assisted stretch. Attempting to lift arm off ball adds a strengthening exercise.*

Date_____ Name_____

Active Assisted Horizontal Abduction 7:4

Starting Position: Kneel behind ball and place one hand on top of ball.

Movement/Exercise: Lean trunk forward and roll ball out to side with straight arm as far as comfort allows. Return to start and repeat to other side.

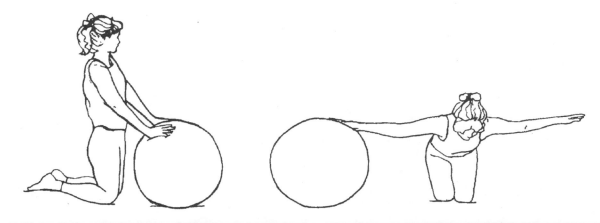

CAUTION: STAY WITHIN PAIN FREE RANGE.

Breathing: Do not hold breath. Breathe comfortably.

Modification:
1. Sit in chair with ball in front on a bed or table.
2. If range is limited, attempt to lift arm off ball at end range.

Progression:
1. Lift arm at end range for isometric strengthening.
2. Add internal and external rotation of shoulder by
    rolling ball forward and backward.

Hold_____Seconds

Repeat_____ Times

Do_____Times/day

Purpose/ Goal:_____

_____

Comments: *The ball supports the weight of the arm as it rolls out to the side. Flexing the trunk forward adds a gravity assisted movement and a comfortable stretch which can be maintained. Attempting to lift arm off ball adds a strengthening exercise.*

Date_____   Name_____

Active Shoulder Horizontal Abduction   7:5

Starting Position: Lie stomach over ball with hands and knees on floor.

Movement/Exercise: Leave injured arm on floor. Press hand into floor and straighten elbow. Lift other arm out to side and allow trunk to twist until fingers point toward ceiling. Eyes should follow lifting hand and weight will be shifted onto support arm.

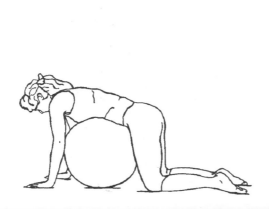 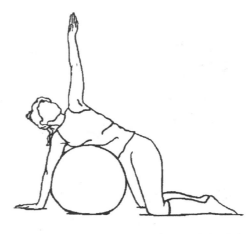

CAUTION: *STAY WITHIN PAIN FREE RANGE.*

Breathing: Inhale while lifting, exhale while returning.

Modification: Shoulder and elbow can be stabilized by an assistant.

Progression:
1. Straighten knees and balance on toes.
2. Lift opposite leg.
3. Lift weight or pull resistive band with upper hand.

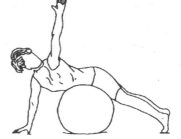

Hold_____Seconds

Weights_____

Repeat_____ Times

Do_____Times/day

Purpose/ Goal:_____

_____

Comments: *The farther the twist, the more weight is put on support arm and shoulder girdle muscles which are coactivated around the joints to increase stability.*

Date_____   Name_____

Internal/External Shoulder Rotation (Single arm)   7:6

Starting Position: Kneel behind ball with one hand on top of ball. Touch fingers of other hand on floor next to hips.

Movement/Exercise: Allowing trunk to follow, roll ball from side to side. Return to center. Switch arms.

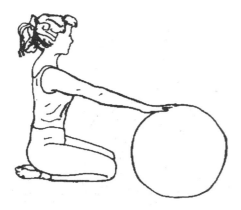 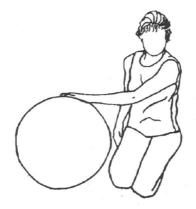

CAUTION: STAY WITHIN PAIN FREE RANGE.

Breathing: Do not hold breath. Breathe comfortably.

Modification:
1. If weakness exists, support/guide arm on ball with other arm.
2. If unable to kneel, sit in chair with ball on bed in front.

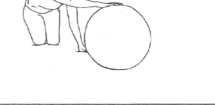

Progression: To add shoulder flexion, lean trunk forward allowing head to fall next to arm and roll ball from side to side.

Hold_____Seconds

Repeat_____ Times

Do_____Times/day

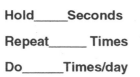

Purpose/ Goal:_____

_____

Comments: *The ball allows precise control of gravity assisted internal and external rotation. It also provides gentle side bending and rotation of the spine.*

Date_____   Name_____

Internal/External Shoulder Rotation (Both arms)   7:7

Starting Position: Sit on heels behind ball with hands shoulder-width apart on ball.

Movement/Exercise: Roll ball in half circle allowing top arm to cross over lower arm. Reverse in other direction.

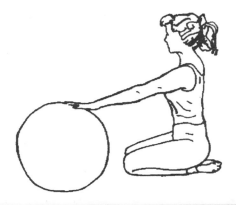 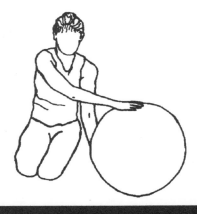

CAUTION: STAY WITHIN PAIN FREE RANGE.

Breathing: Do not hold breath. Breathe comfortably.

Modification: If unable to kneel, sit in chair with ball in front on bed or table.

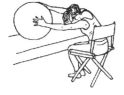

Progression: To combine internal and external rotation with shoulder flexion, roll ball away from body so that trunk lowers and head is between arms.

Hold_____Seconds

Repeat_____ Times

Do_____Times/day

Purpose/ Goal:_____

_____

Comments: *The ball allows precise control of gravity assisted internal and external rotation.*

© 1995 by Joanne Posner-Mayer, PT

Chapter 8 — Standing

Date_____ Name_____

Ball Forward-Standing   8:1

Starting Position: Stand in optimal posture with feet hip-width apart. Hold ball in front with elbows bent at a 90º angle. Tighten abdominal muscles to stabilize low back.

Movement/Exercise: Push ball forward until arms are straight. Reverse and return to start. Repeat.

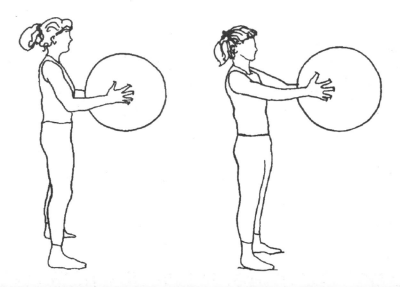

CAUTION: *STAY WITHIN PAIN-FREE RANGE. TIGHTEN TRUNK MUSCLES. DO NOT ALLOW SPINE TO CURVE OR ARCH WITH MOVEMENT.*

Breathing: Inhale as ball is pushed forward, exhale as ball returns.

Modification:
1. Only move arms as far as comfort allows.
2. Step one foot slightly forward to widen base of support for balance assistance.

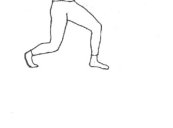

Progression: Combine with stepping one foot forward and backward or walking in tempo with arm movement.

Beats/min_____   Repeat_____ Times   Do_____Times/day

Purpose/ Goal:_____

_____

Comments: *The 55cm ball weighs 1 1/2lbs, the 65cm ball weighs 2lbs. This activates shoulder adductor muscles as well as shoulder flexors and trunk stabilizers. It can also increase cardiovascular output compared to just lifting empty arms.*

Squat Ball Forward-Standing   8:2

Starting Position: Stand in optimal posture with feet hip-width apart. Hold ball in front with elbows flexed at 90 degrees. Tighten abdominal muscles to stabilize spine.

Movement/Exercise: Push ball forward until arms are straight while bending hips and knees. Reverse and return to start. Repeat.

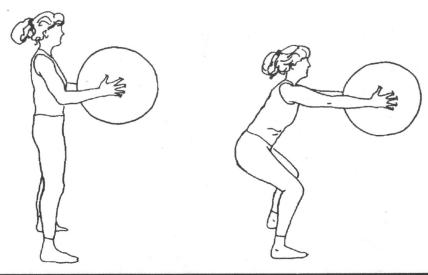

CAUTION: *STAY WITHIN PAIN-FREE RANGE. TIGHTEN TRUNK MUSCLES AND DO NOT ALLOW SPINE TO CURVE OR ARCH WITH MOVEMENT.*

Breathing: Inhale as ball is pushed forward, exhale as ball returns.

Modification:
1. Only move arms as far as comfort allows.
2. Step one foot slightly forward to widen base of support for balance assistance.

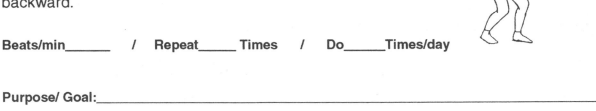

Progression: Combine with stepping one foot forward and backward.

Beats/min_____ / Repeat_____ Times / Do_____Times/day

Purpose/ Goal:_____

_____

Comments: *The 55cm ball weighs 1 1/2lbs, the 65cm ball weighs 2lbs. This activates shoulder adductor muscles as well as shoulder flexors and trunk stabilizers. It can increase cardiovascular output compared to just lifting empty arms. This also trains bending at the hips instead of rounding spine to reach and lift.*

Date_____   Name_____

Ball Overhead-Standing   8:3

Starting Position: Stand with feet hip-width apart. Hold ball in front with elbows flexed at 90º angle. Tighten abdominal muscles to stabilize spine.

Movement/Exercise: Lift ball over head toward ceiling. Lower to start. Repeat.

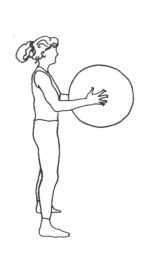 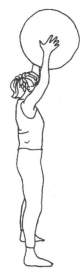 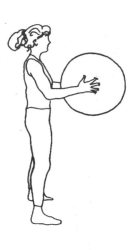

CAUTION: STAY WITHIN PAIN-FREE RANGE. TIGHTEN TRUNK MUSCLES AND DO NOT ALLOW TRUNK TO SWAY WITH MOVEMENT.

Breathing: Inhale while lifting, exhale while lowering.

Modification:
1. Only move arms as far as comfort allows.
2. Step one foot slightly forward for balance assistance.

Progression: Combine with walking around**.**

Beats/min_____

Repeat_____ Times

Do_____Times/day

Purpose/ Goal:_____

_____

Comments: *The 55cm ball weighs 1 1/2lbs, the 65cm balls weighs 2lbs. This activates shoulder adductor muscles as well as shoulder flexors and trunk stabilizers. It can increase cardiovascular output compared to just lifting arms.*

Date_____ Name_____

Marching-Standing 8:4

Starting Position: Stand with feet hip-width apart. Hold ball in front with elbows flexed at a 90° angle. Tighten abdominal muscles to stabilize hips.

Movement/Exercise: Lift ball over head toward ceiling and pick up knees one at a time. Lower ball and leg and repeat with other leg.

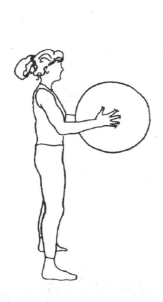 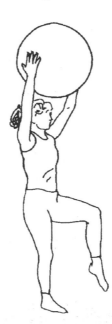

CAUTION: *STAY WITHIN PAIN-FREE RANGE. TIGHTEN TRUNK MUSCLES AND DO NOT ALLOW TRUNK TO SWAY WITH MOVEMENT.*

Breathing: Inhale while lifting, exhale while lowering.

Modification: Only move arms and legs as far as comfort allows.

Progression: Combine with marching forward, backward and sideways.

Beats/min_____

Repeat_____ Times   Do_____Times/day

Purpose/ Goal:_____

_____

Comments: *The 55cm ball weighs 1 1/2lbs, the 65cm ball weighs 2lbs. This activates shoulder adductor muscles as well as shoulder flexors and trunk stabilizers. It can increase cardiovascular output compared to just lifting empty arms. Lifting knee increases time spent balancing on one leg while moving.*

Date_____ Name_____

Ball Sideways-Standing 8:5

Starting Position: Stand with feet hip-width apart. Hold ball in front with elbows extended. Tighten abdominal muscles to stabilize hips.

Movement/Exercise: Keeping trunk still, move ball to one side of body allowing weight to shift to that leg and other heel to come off floor. Return to center. Alternate to other side. Repeat.

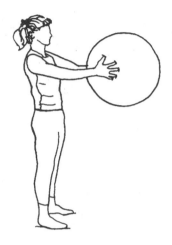 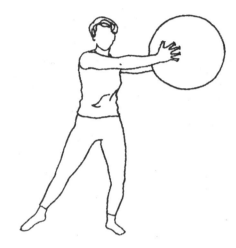

CAUTION: *STAY WITHIN PAIN-FREE RANGE. TIGHTEN TRUNK MUSCLES.*

Breathing: Inhale as ball moves to side, exhale as ball returns to center.

Modification:
1. Only move arms as far as comfort allows.
2. Keep feet flat on floor and do not allow trunk to sway.

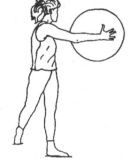

Progression: Allow trunk to twist so that ball moves behind body and head follows ball.

Beats/min_____

Repeat_____ Times   Do_____Times/day

Purpose/ Goal:_____

_____

Comments: *The 55cm ball weighs 1 1/2lbs, the 65cm ball weighs 2lbs. This activates shoulder adductor muscles as well as shoulder flexors and trunk stabilizers. It can increase cardiovascular output compared to just lifting empty arms. Shifting weight from leg to leg adds momentum and velocity and challenges the body's ability to sway and recover.*

Date_____   **Name**_____

Half Squat and Lift-Standing   *8:6*

Starting Position: Keeping spine in optimal posture, push ball forward until arms are straight while bending knees and hips to counterbalance weight. Tighten abdominal muscles to stabilize hips.

Movement/Exercise: Hold squatting position and lift ball overhead and return. Hold, lower ball in front. Repeat or return to start. Repeat.

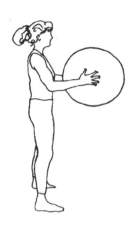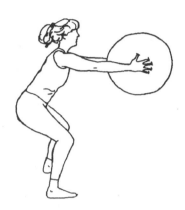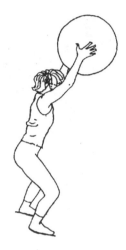

CAUTION: *STAY WITHIN PAIN-FREE RANGE. TIGHTEN TRUNK MUSCLES. MAKE SURE KNEES STAY IN LINE OVER TOES.*

Breathing: Inhale as ball is pushed forward, exhale as ball returns.

Modification:
1. Squat only as far as comfort allows and do not straighten arms.
2. Step one foot slightly forward for balance assist.

Progression: Walk forward and backward stepping in tempo to raising and lowering ball.

Beats/min_____

Repeat_____ **Times**   **Do**_____**Times/day**

Purpose/ Goal:_____

_____

Comments: *The 55cm ball weighs 1 1/2lbs, the 65cm ball weighs 2lbs. Besides activating the shoulder girdle and trunk stabilizers, this exercise strengthens the muscles of the legs and spine used in functional lifting patterns.*

© 1995 by Joanne Posner-Mayer, PT

Date_____   Name_____

Squat and Lift-Standing   8:7

Starting Position: Stand with feet spread about two feet apart and with toes pointing slightly outward. Hold ball in front with elbows bent at a 90° angle. Tighten abdominal muscles to stabilize hips.

Movement/Exercise: Bend hips and knees and lower ball. Then, lift ball towards ceiling while straightening hips and knees.

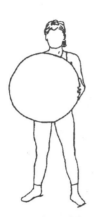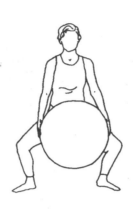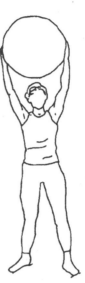

CAUTION: *STAY WITHIN PAIN-FREE RANGE. TIGHTEN TRUNK MUSCLES AND DO NOT ALLOW TRUNK TO SWAY WITH MOVEMENT. MAKE SURE KNEES STAY IN LINE OVER TOES.*

Breathing: Inhale while lifting, exhale while lowering.

Modification: Only squat and/or move arms as far as comfort allows.

Progression: As ball is raised overhead and hips and knees straighten, raise up on toes.

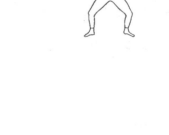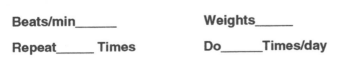

Beats/min_____   Weights_____

Repeat_____ Times   Do_____Times/day

Purpose/ Goal:_____

_____

Comments: *The 55cm ball weighs 1 1/2lbs, the 65cm ball weighs 2lbs. Besides activating the shoulder girdle and trunk stabilizers, this exercise strengthens the muscles of the legs used in functional lifting patterns. It challenges balance by decreasing the base of support and increasing the lever arm.*

Date_____   Name_____

Side Bend-Standing   8:8

Starting Position: Stand with feet spread about two feet apart and with toes pointing slightly outward. Hold ball between one arm and side of trunk. Raise other arm out to side parallel to floor.

Movement/Exercise: Raise free arm up toward ceiling and simultaneously side bend trunk letting weight rest on ball while hips sway to opposite side for counter balance. Hold. Return to start. Repeat. Switch to other side.

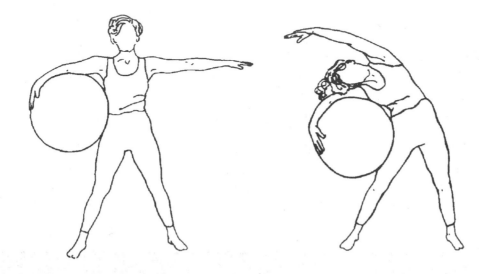

CAUTION: STAY WITHIN PAIN-FREE RANGE. KEEP KNEES IN LINE WITH TOES.

Breathing: Inhale while side bending, exhale while returning to start.

Modification: Only bend as far as comfort allows or keep opposite arm at side.

Progression: Push up on toe on side of ball causing increased trunk sway and side bend.

Repeat_____ Times   /   Do_____ Times/day

Purpose/ Goal:_____

_____

Comments: *This is a gravity-assisted side bending stretch to increase flexibility of spine and ribs and can increase respiratory capacity on inhalation. Sway challenges balance.*

Date_____   Name_____

Toss and Catch-Standing   8:9

Starting Position: Stand with feet spread about two feet apart and allow toes to point outward. Hold ball in front with elbows bent at 90º. Bend hips and knees slightly. Tighten abdominal muscles to stabilize hips.

Movement/Exercise: Straighten hips and knees as arms toss ball against wall. As ball is caught, allow hips and knees to bend.

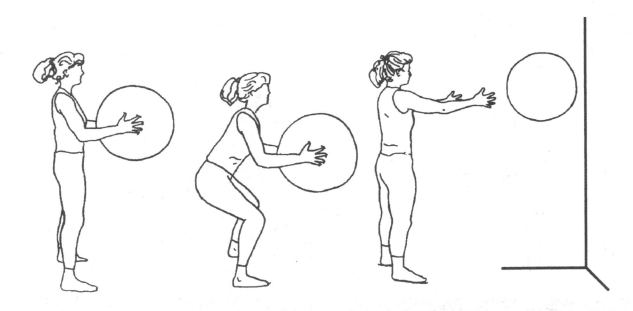

CAUTION: *STAY WITHIN PAIN-FREE RANGE. MAKE SURE KNEES STAY IN LINE OVER TOES.*

Breathing: Inhale as ball is thrown, exhale as ball is caught.

Modification: Keep hips and knees straight as ball is tossed and caught.

Progression: Raise up on toes as ball is tossed, return heels to floor as ball is caught.

Beats/min_____

Repeat_____ Times   Do_____Times/day

Purpose/ Goal:_____

_____

Comments: The 55cm ball weighs 1 1/2lbs, the 65cm ball weighs 2lbs. Catching the ball requires trunk stabilizers to activate and absorb the momentum of tossing and catching the ball to maintain balance.

© 1995 by Joanne Posner-Mayer PT

Date_____   Name_____

Wall Squat-Body Mechanics   8:10

Starting Position: Stand with feet spread hip width apart and toes pointing forward with back to wall. Place ball between back and wall. Be sure not to lean backward against ball. Tighten abdominal muscles to stabilize hips. Pretend there is a box in front of feet.

Movement/Exercise: Bending hips and knees, lower body as if to pick up box. Ball will roll up back assisting trunk to lean forward as hips hinge backward to simulate proper body mechanics for lifting. Hold. Straighten hips and knees to return to start.

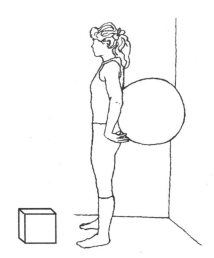 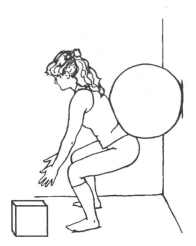

CAUTION: *STAY WITHIN PAIN-FREE RANGE. KEEP KNEES IN LINE WITH TOES AND FEET FLAT ON FLOOR WHILE MAINTAINING SPINE IN OPTIMAL ALIGNMENT. DO NOT SLANT BODY BACKWARDS.*

Breathing: Exhale while squatting, inhale while returning to standing position.

Modification: Only squat as far as comfort allows.

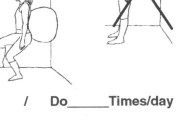

Progression:
1. Hold weighted ball or free weights in hands.
2. Pick up one leg and squat as far as balance allows.

Beats/min_____ / Weights_____ / Repeat_____ Times / Do_____Times/day

Purpose/ Goal:_____

_____

Comments: *This provides eccentric and concentric quadriceps and gluteal muscle strengthening while teaching proper body mechanics for squatting.*

Name_____   Date_____

Glide-Extra Credit   8:11

Starting Position: Sit on ball in optimal posture.

Movement/Exercise: Step out to side with right foot and touch toes of left foot in front of it. Touch left hand to ball and raise right arm. Reverse by taking a big step out with left foot. Cross toes of right foot in front of left foot while reversing arms.

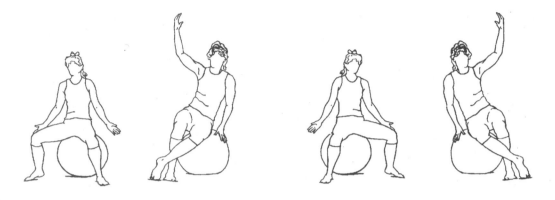

CAUTION: *ONLY GO AS FAST AS BALANCE ALLOWS. START SLOWLY. GET MOVEMENTS SYNCHRONIZED BEFORE ADVANCING.*

Breathing: Breathe comfortably. Do not hold breath.

Modification: Have someone guard by standing behind and give balance support by holding waist.

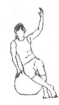

Progression:
1. Lift both feet at the same time and switch feet in air as ball rolls underneath buttocks.
2. Stand up at the end of each movement to the side with hand touching ball.
3. Add speed.

Beats/min_____

Repeat_____ Times

Do_____Times/day

Purpose/ Goal:_____

_____

Comments: *Absorption of momentum challenges balance, timing, coordination and proprioception.*

Date_____   Name_____

Kneel Stand-Extra Credit   *8:12*

Starting Position: Assume Total Body Flexion position (exercise 5:6).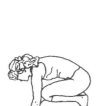

Movement/Exercise: Master each step before advancing.
1. Rise until only fingertips touch floor for balance.
2. Remove fingers from floor to free arms for balancing.
3. Raise trunk slowly to upright.
4. Straighten hips and knees rising to kneeling position. Hold for as long as balance allows.
5. To dismount-roll ball backward and let feet touch floor until standing.

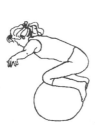 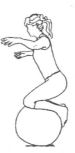 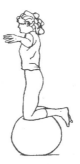 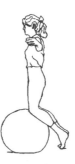

CAUTION: *DO EXERCISE IN LARGE AREA CLEAR OF OBJECTS. PROVIDE ENOUGH UNOBSTRUCTED SPACE TO PREVENT COLLISION. IF BALL ROLLS FORWARD, BE PREPARED TO BEND AT WAIST AND PUT HANDS ON FLOOR.*

Breathing: Breathe comfortably. Do not hold breath.

Modification: Touch someone or some stable object lightly for balance assistance.

Progression: Once upright, move arms in random motion to challenge balance or do aerobic arm movements, golf, tennis, pitching, etc...

Beats/min_____   /   Repeat_____ Times   /   Do_____Times/day

Purpose/ Goal:_____

_____

Comments: *This exercise raises the center of gravity of the body higher than usual and forces it to balance on an unstable base of support. This challenges balance beyond normal levels required for upright function. However, it can be very useful to improve balance skill level for sports and other demanding work situations.*

Chapter 9   Resistive Band

Resistive Band Exercises

Resistive band is a very effective tool for strengthening exercises. Any exercise that is done with resistive band while sitting in a chair can be done while sitting on the ball.

Keep wrists in neutral alignment. Do not allow wrists to move as resistive band stretches.

If not properly held, it can slip from hands. To avoid this choose one of the following:

1. Tie knots in each end.

2. Grasp each end in palm of hand with palms down and then twist band once around hand.

3. Loop resistive band in half and tie both ends together in one knot.

4. Fit ends into handles or tie to Gym Rings.

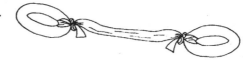

* Before adding resistive band:
Try all exercises to establish pain free range of motion and strength against gravity.

Date_____ Name_____

Resistive Band Shoulder Horizontal Abduction   9:1

Starting Position: Sit on ball in optimal posture. Properly grasp resistive band. Raise arms out in front with arms shoulders' width apart. Tighten abdominal muscles.

Movement/Exercise: Open arms out to side stretching resistive band. Slowly reverse so that band remains taut at all times. Repeat.

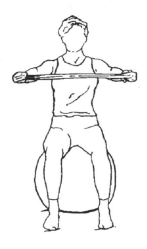 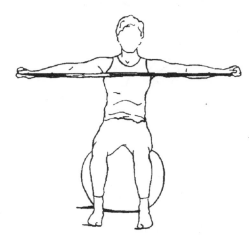

CAUTION: *STAY WITHIN PAIN FREE RANGE. KEEP WRISTS IN NEUTRAL ALIGNMENT. DO NOT ALLOW WRISTS TO MOVE AS RESISTIVE BAND STRETCHES.*

Breathing: Inhale as band stretches, exhale on return.

Modification:
1. Lower arms.
2. Move only one arm at a time.

Progression: Pick one foot up off ground and/or close eyes.

Hold_____Seconds

Repeat_____ Times

Do_____Times/day

Purpose/ Goal:_____

_____

Comments: The ball creates a mobile base of support as resistive band is stretched and challenges the muscles that provide lower extremity and spinal stabilization. Feel shoulder blades adduct as band is stretched. Decreasing base of support increases difficulty.

Date_____ **Name**_____

Resistive Band Shoulder Flexion to Abduction　9:2

Starting Position: Sit on ball in optimal posture. Properly grasp resistive band. Raise straight arms overhead a shoulders' width apart. Tighten abdominal muscles.

Movement/Exercise: Stretch resistive band by letting arms lower out to sides at shoulder level as resistive band lowers behind head. Slowly reverse. Repeat.

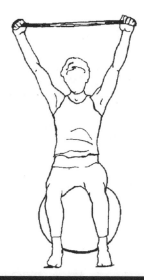 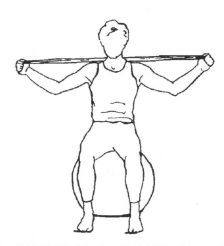

CAUTION: *STAY WITHIN PAIN FREE RANGE. KEEP WRISTS IN NEUTRAL ALIGNMENT. DO NOT ALLOW WRISTS TO MOVE AS RESISTIVE BAND STRETCHES.*

Breathing: Inhale as band stretches, exhale on return.

Modification:
1. Only lower arms as far as comfort allows.
2. Only move one arm at a time.

Progression: Pick one foot up off ground and/or close eyes.

Hold_____**Seconds**

Repeat_____ **Times**

Do_____**Times/day**

Purpose/ Goal:_____

_____

Comments: *The ball creates a mobile base of support as band is stretched and challenges the muscles that provide lower extremity and spinal stabilization while also strengthening shoulder girdle muscles.*

Date_____   Name_____

Resistive Band Elbow Extension Forward   9:3

Starting Position: Sit on ball in optimal posture. Properly grasp resistive band. Put it around shoulders with hands in front of shoulder joints. Tighten abdominal muscles.

Movement/Exercise: Straighten arms forward at shoulder height. Slowly reverse so that band remains taut at all times. Repeat.

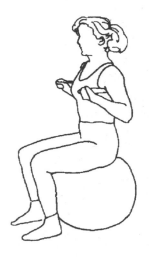 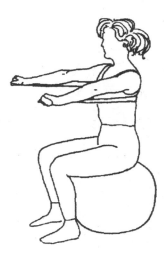

CAUTION: *STAY WITHIN PAIN FREE RANGE. KEEP WRISTS IN NEUTRAL ALIGNMENT. DO NOT ALLOW WRISTS TO MOVE AS RESISTIVE BAND STRETCHES.*

Breathing: Inhale as band stretches, exhale on return.

Modification: Extend one arm at a time.

Progression: Pick one foot up off ground and/or close eyes.

Hold _____Seconds

Repeat_____ Times

Do_____Times/day

Purpose/ Goal:_____

_____

Comments: The ball creates a mobile base of support as band is stretched and challenges the muscles that provide lower extremity and spinal stabilization. Decreasing base of support increases difficulty.

Date_____   Name_____

Resistive Band Shoulder and Elbow Extension   9:4

Starting Position: Sit on ball in optimal posture. Double band into loop. Grasp ends with one hand at opposite shoulder. Put other hand in loop. Tighten abdominal muscles.

Movement/Exercise: Straighten elbow and press arm behind trunk stretching band until arm is straightened as far back as possible. Slowly reverse so that band remains taut at all times. Repeat. Switch to other side.

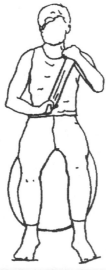 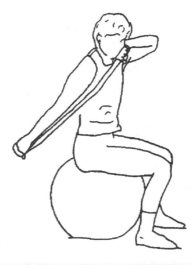

CAUTION: *STAY WITHIN PAIN FREE RANGE. KEEP WRIST IN NEUTRAL ALIGNMENT. DO NOT ALLOW WRISTS TO MOVE AS RESISTIVE BAND STRETCHES.*

Breathing: Inhale as band stretches, exhale on return.

Modification: Only straighten elbow as far as comfort allows.

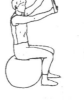 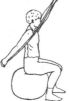

Progression:
1. Hold both arms out in front, pull one arm down past side and behind body.
2. Pick one foot up off ground and/or close eyes.

Hold _____Seconds   Repeat_____ Times   Do_____Times/day

Purpose/ Goal:_____

_____

Comments: *The ball creates a mobile base of support as band is stretched and challenges the muscles that provide lower extremity and spinal stabilization. Feel shoulder blade adduct as arm is extended backward. Decreasing base of support increases difficulty.*

© 1995 by Joanne Posner-Mayer, PT

Date_____ Name_____

Resistive Band Elbow Flexion 9:5

Starting Position: Sit on ball in optimal posture. Properly grasp resistive band. Place it under thighs. Place hands at thigh level. Tighten abdominal muscles.

Movement/Exercise: Bend elbows by bringing hands up to shoulder level. Slowly reverse so that band remains taut at all times. Repeat.

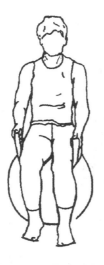 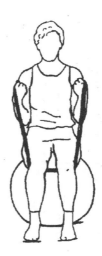

CAUTION: *STAY WITHIN PAIN FREE RANGE. KEEP WRISTS IN NEUTRAL ALIGNMENT. DO NOT ALLOW WRISTS TO MOVE AS RESISTIVE BAND STRETCHES.*

Breathing: Inhale as band stretches, exhale on return.

Modification: Move only one arm at a time or only do part of the movement.

Progression:
1. Pick one foot up off ground and/or close eyes.
2. To bend elbows through full range, put band under feet and start with fully straightened elbows.

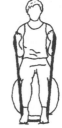

Hold_____Seconds   **Repeat_____ Times**

Do_____Times/day

Purpose/ Goal:_____

_____

Comments: The ball creates a mobile base of support as band is stretched and challenges the muscles that provide lower extremity and spinal stabilization. Decreasing base of support increases difficulty.

Date_____   Name_____

Starting Position: Sit on ball in optimal posture. Properly hold each end of band with each hand. Place hands on opposite knees.

Movement/Exercise: Lift and straighten one arm overhead until upper arm is next to ear. Slowly reverse so that band remains taut at all times. Repeat. Alternate arms.

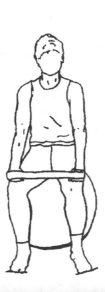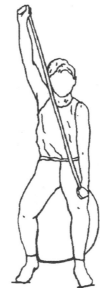

CAUTION: *STAY WITHIN PAIN FREE RANGE. KEEP WRISTS IN NEUTRAL ALIGNMENT. DO NOT ALLOW WRISTS TO MOVE AS RESISTIVE BAND STRETCHES.*

Breathing: Inhale as band stretches, exhale on return.

Modification: Only move arm as far as comfort allows.

Progression: Pick one foot up off ground and/or close eyes.

Hold_____Seconds   Repeat _____ Times

Do_____Times/day

Purpose/ Goal:_____

_____

Comments: *The ball creates a mobile base of support as resistive band is stretched and challenges the muscles that provide lower extremity and spinal stabilization. Decreasing base of support increases difficulty.*

Resistive Band Shoulder Abduction
9:7

Starting Position: Sit on ball in optimal posture. Properly grasp resistive band. Place it under one thigh with one hand between legs. Tighten abdominal muscles.

Movement/Exercise: Lift outside arm out to side and up as high as possible, keeping elbow straight. Slowly reverse so that band remains taut at all times. Repeat. Switch to other side.

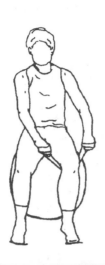
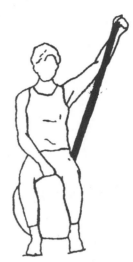

CAUTION: *STAY WITHIN PAIN FREE RANGE. KEEP WRISTS IN NEUTRAL ALIGNMENT. DO NOT ALLOW WRISTS TO MOVE AS RESISTIVE BAND STRETCHES.*

Breathing: Inhale as band stretches, exhale on return.

Modification: Only lift arm to shoulder level or as far as comfort allows.

Progression:
1. Pick one foot up off ground and/or close eyes.
2. Place band under opposite foot.

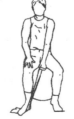
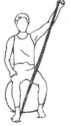

Hold_____Seconds   Repeat_____ Times

Do_____Times/day

Purpose/ Goal:_____

_____

Comments: The ball creates a mobile base of support as band is stretched and challenges the muscles that provide lower extremity and spinal stabilization. Decreasing base of support increases difficulty.

Date_____   Name_____

Resistive Band Chop and Lift   9:8

Starting Position: Sit on ball in optimal posture. Place band under one foot and properly grasp other end with opposite hand. Grab wrist with other hand waist high. Tighten abdominal muscles.

Movement/Exercise: With straight arm, pull band from waist level up and across body ending overhead. Eyes can follow hands while keeping spine still. Reverse slowly keeping band taut at all times. Repeat. Switch to other side.

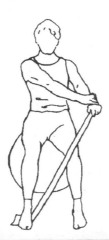 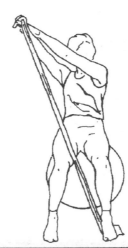

CAUTION: *STAY WITHIN PAIN FREE RANGE. KEEP WRISTS IN NEUTRAL ALIGNMENT. DO NOT ALLOW WRISTS TO MOVE AS RESISTIVE BAND STRETCHES.*

Breathing: Inhale as band stretches, exhale on return.

Modification: Do one arm at a time.

Progression:
1. Allow trunk to join in movement instead of keeping spine still. Bend over to start and straighten hips and trunk up to lift.
2. Allow ball to roll backward while flexing and forward while lifting.
3. Use only one hand to lift as per progressions 1 & 2.

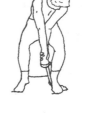

Hold _____Seconds   Repeat_____ Times   Do_____Times/day

Purpose/ Goal:_____

_____

Comments: *The ball creates a mobile base of support as band is stretched and challenges the muscles that provide lower extremity and spinal stabilization while strengthening shoulder flexors.*

Date_____   Name_____

Resistive Band Hip Abduction 9:9

Starting Position: Sit on ball in optimal posture. Wrap band around thighs and properly hold it with one or both hands.

Movement/Exercise: Step one leg out at a time. Slowly reverse so that band remains taut at all times. Repeat. Alternate legs.

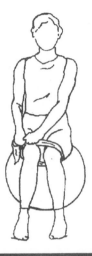 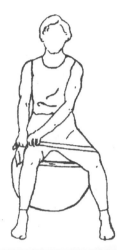

CAUTION: *STAY WITHIN PAIN FREE RANGE. KEEP WRISTS IN NEUTRAL ALIGNMENT. DO NOT ALLOW WRISTS TO MOVE AS RESISTIVE BAND STRETCHES.*

Breathing: Inhale as band stretches, exhale on return.

Modification: Open knees while keeping feet still on floor.

Progression: Keep stepping foot up off ground as it opens and closes and/or close eyes.

Hold _____Seconds   /   Repeat_____ Times   /   Do_____Times/day

Purpose/ Goal:_____

_____

Comments: *The ball creates a mobile base of support as resistive band is stretched and challenges the muscles that provide lower extremity and spinal stabilization. Moving leg continually changes the center of gravity over the base of support. Decreasing base of support increases difficulty.*

Date_____   Name_____

Resistive Band Knee Flexion/Hip Extension   9:10

Starting Position: Sit on ball in optimal posture. Properly grasp resistive band. Place band around one foot.

Movement/Exercise: Keeping hands still at sides. Straighten knee and hip until foot is out in front. Slowly bend hip and knee so that band remains taut at all times. Repeat. Switch legs.

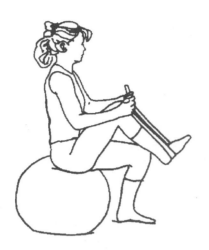
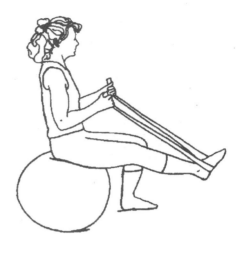

CAUTION: *STAY WITHIN PAIN FREE RANGE. KEEP WRISTS IN NEUTRAL ALIGNMENT. DO NOT ALLOW WRISTS TO MOVE AS RESISTIVE BAND STRETCHES.*

Breathing: Inhale as band stretches, exhale on return.

Modification: Touch hands to ball while holding band for balance assist.

Progression: Close eyes to increase proprioceptive input and challenge balance.

Hold_____Seconds

Repeat_____ Times

Do_____Times/day

Purpose/ Goal:_____

_____

Comments: The ball creates a mobile base of support as resistive band is stretched and challenges the muscles that provide lower extremity and spinal stabilization. Moving leg continually changes the center of gravity over the base of support. Decreasing base of support increases difficulty.

Date_____ Name_____

Resistive Band Prone Shoulder Flexion   9:11

Starting Position: Kneel prone over ball. Properly hold each end of the band with both hands placed on floor. Keeping elbows straight, put weight on one hand.

Movement/Exercise: Lift straight arm overhead until upper arm is next to ear. Slowly reverse so that band remains taut at all times. Repeat. Alternate arms.

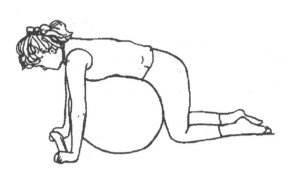 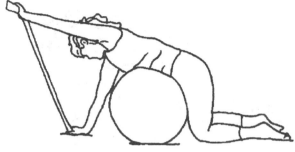

CAUTION: *STAY WITHIN PAIN FREE RANGE. KEEP WRISTS IN NEUTRAL ALIGNMENT. DO NOT ALLOW WRISTS TO DEVIATE AS RESISTIVE BAND STRETCHES.*

Breathing: Inhale as band stretches, exhale on return.

Modification: Only move arm as far as comfort allows.

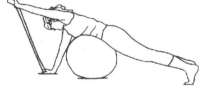

Progression:
1. Dig toes into the floor and straighten knees.
2. Pick one foot up off ground.
3. Lift other arm off floor alongside hip.

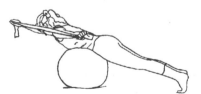

Hold_____Seconds

Repeat _____ Times

Do_____Times/day

Purpose/ Goal:_____

_____

Comments: The ball creates a mobile base of support as resistive band is stretched and challenges the muscles that provide spinal and extremity stabilization. Feel shoulder blade adduct toward spine as arm is lifted. Decreasing base of support increases difficulty.

Date_____   **Name**_____

Resistive Band Prone Shoulder Extension   *9:12*

Starting Position: Lie prone over ball. Wrap band around wrists and properly hold it with both hands. Keeping elbows straight, put weight on one hand on floor.

Movement/Exercise: Raise other arm up alongside hip so that arm is parallel with the floor as band stretches. Slowly reverse so that band remains taut at all times. Repeat. Alternate arms.

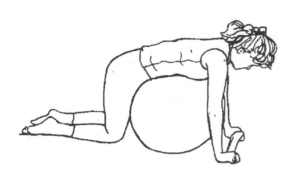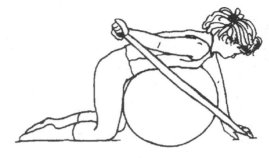

CAUTION: *STAY WITHIN PAIN FREE RANGE. KEEP WRISTS IN NEUTRAL ALIGNMENT. DO NOT ALLOW WRISTS TO DEVIATE AS RESISTIVE BAND STRETCHES.*

Breathing: Inhale as band stretches, exhale on return.

Modification: Only move arm as far as comfort allows. Place knuckles on floor and keep wrist straight.

Progression:
1. Lift both arms next to head and parallel to floor. Pull one arm down towards floor then up alongside hip.
2. Dig toes into the floor and straighten knees while performing exercise.
3. Perform as above and pick one foot up off ground.

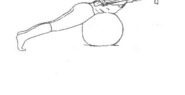

Hold _____ **Seconds**

Repeat _____ **Times**

Do _____ **Times/day**

Purpose/ Goal:_____

_____

Comments: The ball creates a mobile base of support as resistive band is stretched and challenges the muscles that provide spinal and extremity stabilization. Feel shoulder blade adduct toward spine as arm is lifted. Decreasing base of support increases difficulty.

Date_____   Name_____

Resistive Band Prone Shoulder Abduction   9:13

Starting Position: Lie prone over ball. Wrap resistive band around wrists and properly hold it with each hand. Place hands on floor. Keeping elbows straight, put weight on one hand.

Movement/Exercise: Raise opposite arm out to side so that arm is parallel with floor as band stretches. Reverse slowly keeping band taut at all times. Repeat. Alternate arms.

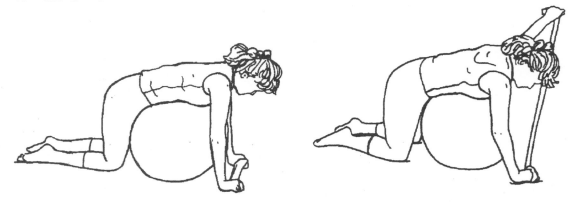

CAUTION: *STAY WITHIN PAIN FREE RANGE. KEEP WRISTS IN NEUTRAL ALIGNMENT. DO NOT ALLOW WRISTS TO MOVE AS RESISTIVE BAND STRETCHES.*

Breathing: Inhale as band stretches, exhale on return.

Modification: Only move arm as far as comfort allows. Place knuckles on floor and keep wrist straight.

Progression:
1. Dig toes into the floor and straighten knees.
2. Pick one foot up off ground.
3. Raise both arms up off floor and either abduct one arm at a time or both arms simultaneously.

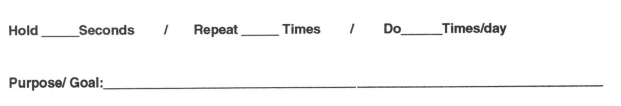

Hold _____Seconds   /   Repeat _____ Times   /   Do_____Times/day

Purpose/ Goal:_____

_____

Comments: The ball creates a mobile base of support as resistive band is stretched and challenges the muscles that provide spinal and extremity stabilization. Feel shoulder blade adduct toward spine as arm are lifted. Decreasing base of support increases difficulty.

Date_____   Name_____

Shoulder Blade Squeeze with Weights   10:1

Starting Position: Kneel behind ball. Lie trunk over ball and grasp weights.

Movement/Exercise: Lift upper arms out to side. Allow elbows to bend and squeeze shoulder blades together. Keep elbows straight out to side at shoulder level. Return to start and repeat.

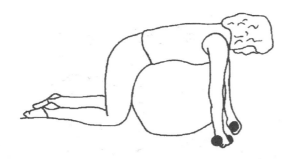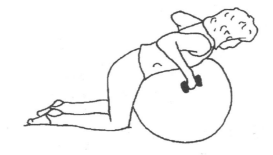

CAUTION: *KEEP NECK STILL IN OPTIMAL POSITION WITH EYES FOCUSED ON FLOOR.*

Breathing: Inhale while lifting, exhale on return.

Modification:
1. Lift arms only as far as comfort allows.
2. Lift one arm at a time.

Progression: Dig toes in floor and extend knees.

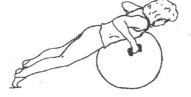

Weights_____

Repeat_____ Times

Do_____Times/day

Purpose/ Goal:_____

_____

Comments: *The ball adds a dynamic base of support to challenge balance while strengthening the shoulder girdle. When legs are straightened, the base of support decreases to further challenge balance and trunk stability.*

Date_____ Name_____

Straight Arm Lifts-Side with Weights   10:2

Starting Position: Kneel behind ball. Lie trunk over ball and grasp weights.

Movement/Exercise: Lift straight arms out to side while squeezing shoulder blades together. Keep arms to side at shoulder level. Return to start and repeat.

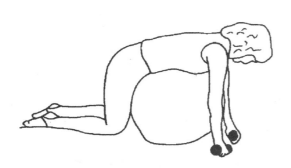 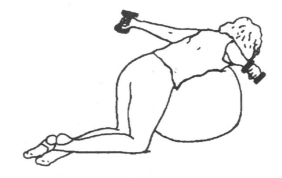

CAUTION: *KEEP NECK STILL IN OPTIMAL POSITION WITH EYES FOCUSED ON FLOOR.*

Breathing: Inhale while lifting, exhale on return.

Modification:
1. Lift arms only as far as comfort allows.
2. Lift one arm at a time.

Progression: Dig toes in floor and straighten knees.

Weights_____

Repeat_____ Times

Do_____Times/day

Purpose/ Goal:_____

_____

Comments: *The ball adds a dynamic base of support to challenge balance while strengthening the shoulder girdle. When legs are straightened, the base of support decreases to further challenge balance and trunk stability while increasing the lever arm.*

Date_____   Name_____

Shoulder Extension with Weights   10:3

Starting Position: Kneel behind ball. Lie trunk on ball and grasp weights.

Movement/Exercise: Keeping elbows straight, lift arms past hips towards ceiling. Return to start and repeat. Palms can face ceiling, floor or body.

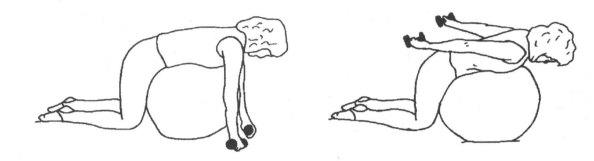

CAUTION: *KEEP NECK IN OPTIMAL POSITION WITH FACE TOWARDS FLOOR.*

Breathing: Inhale while lifting, exhale on return.

Modification:
1. Only lift arms as far as comfort allows.
2. Lift one arm at a time.

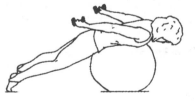

Progression: Dig toes into floor and extend knees.

Weights_____

Repeat_____ Times

Do_____Times/day

Purpose/ Goal:_____

_____

Comments: *Hand position can target various shoulder girdle muscles. The ball adds a dynamic base of support to challenge balance while strengthening the shoulder girdle. When legs are straightened, the base of support decreases to further challenge balance and trunk stability.*

Date_____ **Name**_____

Alternate Arm Lifts with Weights 10:4

Starting Position: Kneel behind ball. Lie trunk on ball and grasp weights.

Movement/Exercise: Keeping elbows straight, simultaneously lift one arm past hip towards ceiling and other arm up along side of head. Lower arms to floor. Repeat. Palms can face ceiling, floor or body.

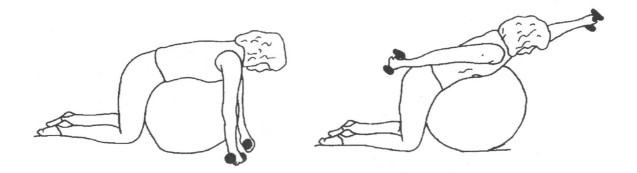

CAUTION: KEEP NECK IN OPTIMAL POSITION WITH FACE TOWARDS FLOOR.

Breathing: Inhale while lifting, exhale on return.

Modification:
1. Only lift arms as far as comfort allows.
2. Only lift one arm at a time.

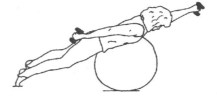

Progression: Dig toes into floor and extend knees.

Weights_____

Repeat_____ **Times**

Do_____**Times/day**

Purpose/ Goal:_____

_____

Comments: *Hand position can target various shoulder girdle muscles. The ball adds a dynamic base of support to challenge balance while strengthening the shoulder girdle. When legs are straightened, the base of support decreases to further challenge balance and trunk stability.*

Date_____ Name_____

Elbow Extension with Weights   10:5

Starting Position: Kneel behind ball. Lie trunk on ball and grasp weights. Lift upper arms out to side. Allow elbows to bend and squeeze shoulder blades together.

Movement/Exercise: Straighten elbows as forearm lifts out to side at shoulder level. Hold. Return to starting position by bending elbows. Repeat. .

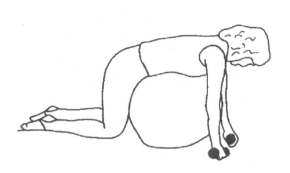 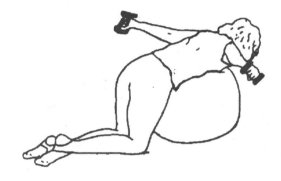

CAUTION: *KEEP NECK IN OPTIMAL POSITION WITH FACE TOWARDS FLOOR.*

Breathing: Inhale while lifting, exhale on return.

Modification:
1. Only lift arms as far as comfort allows.
2. Lift one arm at a time.

Progression: Dig toes into floor and straighten knees.

Weights_____

Repeat _____ Times

Do_____Times/day

Purpose/ Goal:_____

_____

Comments: Hand position can target various shoulder girdle muscles. The ball adds a dynamic base of support to challenge balance while strengthening the shoulder girdle. When legs are straightened, the base of support decreases to further challenge balance and trunk stability.

Date_____   Name_____

Shoulder Flexion with Weights   10:6

Starting Position: Kneel behind ball.   Lie trunk on ball and grasp weights.

Movement/Exercise: Keeping elbows straight, lift both arms up alongside head. Hold. Return to starting position by lowering arms. Repeat.

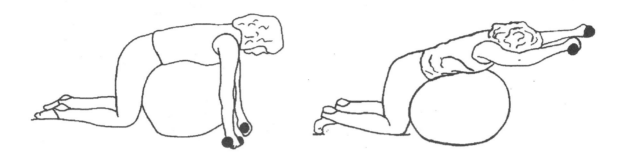

CAUTION: *KEEP NECK IN OPTIMAL POSITION WITH FACE TOWARDS FLOOR.*

Breathing: Inhale while lifting, exhale on return.

Modification:
1. Only lift arms as far as comfort allows.
2. Lift one arm at a time.

Progression: Dig toes into floor and straighten knees.

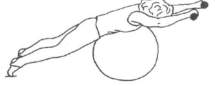

Weights_____

Repeat_____ Times

Do_____Times/day

Purpose/ Goal:_____

_____

Comments: Hand position can target various shoulder girdle muscles. The ball adds a dynamic base of support to challenge balance while strengthening the shoulder girdle. When legs are straightened, the base of support decreases to further challenge balance and trunk stability.

Suggested Inflation Instructions

Before inflating a ball, check for any damage. If the box is crushed during shipment, there is a small possibility that the ball was damaged. Although any damage is uncommon, notify the supplier if there are any questions. Balls should also be inspected before each use for gouges or deep scratches. Do not attempt to repair a ball if it has been punctured or gouged. After repair, the risk of it breaking while in use is more likely and the impact is equivalent to having a chair pulled out from under you. Be sure to check the ball's weight capacity before using it to sit on or for exercising.

There are different brands of balls and the types of plugs may vary. Some use a rubber plug like in a basketball, others use a short plastic plugs. One manufacturer includes a long plug in the ball and a small packet containing another plug and an inflation adapter with a ball bearing in it. The long plug was designed specifically for people using the ball around children. It is very difficult to remove from the ball and is impossible to swallow because of its length. Remove this plug before attempting to inflate the ball. The adapter is made for European bicycle pumps 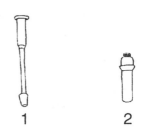 and generally will not work with American pumps. If the smaller, outside thread is cut off, it can be used with American bicycle pumps and at gas stations that do not have adapter nozzles. Do not push this adapter into the ball!

The ball will not properly inflate unless it is at room temperature. The balls require a high volume of air at low pressure. Therefore, a bicycle pump, which produces a low volume of air at high pressure, is not recommended. Electric air compressors and manual air raft or mattress pumps that have a cone shaped nozzle are best. Also, car or tire repair facilities usually have compressed air in their shops. Ask if they have a cone shaped (trigger) nozzle. Use correct body mechanics for back, knees and wrists when using a hand pump to inflate the ball (see Pump Instructions, page 195).

The balls are inflated according to size not pressure. Some of the balls have the maximum diameter (height off the floor) of the ball printed on it. Over inflating the ball will stretch the vinyl too thin and reduce the ball's strength. The ball may be used slightly under inflated but it is recommended that it be large enough so that the hips and knees are bent at 90° angles when sitting on it (Kucera, Klein-Vogelbach). For detailed instructions, see page 26 .

To begin, take a yardstick or tape measure and mark maximum diameter (height) for the ball on a wall or door. Use chosen pump and start pumping air into ball. Put plug in ball and measure the ball by placing a yardstick on top of ball and comparing it with the mark on the wall or door. Add more air as necessary.

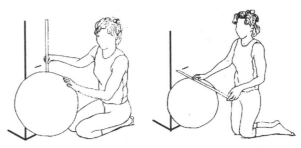

DO NOT INFLATE THE BALL LARGER THAN THE MAXIMUM DIAMETER SPECIFIED

Cleaning and General Instructions

To clean the ball, use a cloth and warm soapy water. Do not use abrasive or chemical cleaners. Standard hospital disinfectants are safe if there is no warning on the label about using them on vinyl (PVC) surfaces.

General Safety Instructions

1. Keep the ball away from sources of heat or direct sunlight for extended periods of time.

2. Check the area and clothing for sharp objects that may puncture the ball.

3. Provide unobstructed space so furniture or other objects that could cause injury are not in the immediate area.

4. Maintain optimal posture while bouncing. **Do not combine bouncing with bending, twisting or rotating the spine.**

5. Perform exercises slowly and with control.

6. A heavy pony tail may cause discomfort to the neck. If so, modify this hair style.

7. Bare feet are recommended when exercising, however, if feet are slipping, rubber soled shoes are advised.

8. When wearing athletic shoes that have been worn outside, check the soles for pebbles. These may fall out of the soles and puncture the ball if it happens to roll over them.

9. Wear comfortable clothes that allow full range of movement. Denim jeans or tight fitting pants are usually too restrictive for exercises. Shorts should be at least knee length as bare skin will often stick to the ball, hinder movement and/or cause discomfort.

Checking for air leakage and punctures

1. If the ball loses air, first check for air escaping through the plug by putting a few drops of water around it. Watch for air bubbles to appear. If air is escaping from plug area, try switching plugs. This usually stops the leakage.

2. If the ball still loses air, check for a gouge or puncture. Inflate the ball until it is firm and take a very wet sponge or cloth and rub over surface of the ball. Listen for the hissing sound of air escaping as it comes in contact with the water. If the ball is punctured, discard and replace it. When pressure (weight) is applied to a punctured ball, the puncture may tear and the ball will collapse. Working on a punctured and/or repaired ball is dangerous and responsibility for resulting injury may fall on therapist/facility/self.

Using the Power Air Pump:

1.   Place one foot (or toes of one foot) on each side of the pump base. Using correct body mechanics (see pictures), bend at hips and knees keeping knees over toes and spine in optimal posture *(a)*. Grasp handle with hands and pull up by straightening knees and hips *(b)*. Push down on handle through straight arms by using body weight and simultaneously bend knees and hips *(a)*.   Keep back stabilized in optimal posture. Repeat. Do not pump by bending back and hips while keeping knees straight or pull on handle by bending and straightening elbows.

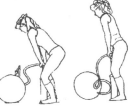

a   b

Using Quick Air Pump:

1.   The pump comes with (1) a collared piece with two nozzles attached, (2) two red, ribbed connecting pieces and (3) three sections of black hose. Connect the hoses by putting a red connector in the end of the first section. Then, slide the next length of hose onto it until the sections are secure against the center of the connector. Repeat this step with the second connector piece and the third length of hose.

2.   Attach the collar piece to the end of the hose. Make sure that the collar is snugly fit into the hose by sliding it to the rim. Then, stack the first nozzle onto the collar. This nozzle is usually small enough to fit in the ball. If it is not, stack the smallest nozzle on top of the first. Finally, connect the other end of the hose onto the spout at the base of the pump. Place the nozzle into the ball.

3.   Place a foot on each side of the pump base at all times (to ensure one side will not break off). Start pumping air into the ball using proper body mechanics and keeping the spine in optimal posture. Inflate the ball to any size below the maximum, but make sure it is inflated no larger than the maximum diameter. As the ball inflates, it will take more pressure to push air into the ball and pumping will become more strenuous. To rest, put the plug in the ball or recruit another person to assist (air will escape through the pump barrel unless rapid pumping is maintained). Be careful not to bend or kink hose so that air flow is cut off.

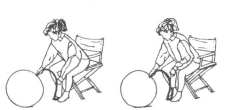

Bellows pumps are not recommended for patient use. As the ball inflates, the pressure necessary to push in air increases and poor body mechanics for back and knees are usually required to force air into the ball.

Follow inflation instructions for proper sizing of the ball (see page 193).

Ball Storage Suggestions

 There are many different ways to store the balls. A Deck, Tennis or Gym Ring can be used as a stand to keep one ball from rolling when not in use. However, if a clinic has several balls, following are some pictures illustrating how some therapists store the balls.

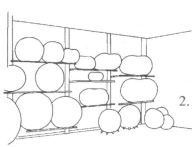

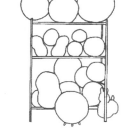

1. Prefabricated washer/dryer rack with middle shelf lowered and shelves turned upside down so that lip is facing upward. Adding the bottom shelf is optional.

2. Prefabricated wire closet rack attached to wall with "L" brackets. The lip has been turned upward to hold balls and rolls more effectively.

 3. Nets can be used to store several balls and hung from the ceiling in a variety of ways.

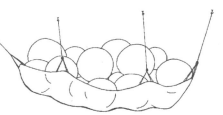

4. For large numbers of balls, a parachute can be purchased at at military surplus store. It can be gathered with sturdy clips (carbiners) and attached to a rope which runs through a pulley system suspended from the ceiling. The parachute illustrated holds over thirty balls.

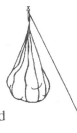

5. Hoops can also be attached to the wall to hold balls off floor. This is a example of a custom made wire hoop rack.

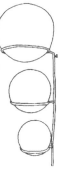

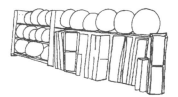

6. Balls and step benches stored on shelving made of metal pipe. The benches are stacked vertically. This is good for aerobic rooms where both types of equipment are used.

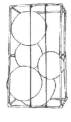

7. PVC sprinkler pipe and connection joints can be assembled to form different cages *(1)* to keep balls on the floor or in a tower *(2)*. With a little creativity, there are also many racks that can be devised using different materials such as wood dowels and elastic tubing. (Tubing keeps balls in and stretches to let balls out.)

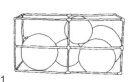

1   2

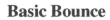

Basic Bounce

Toe Raise

Shoulder Shrug

Tight ArmCircles

Drumming

Arm Swing

Front/Back Clap

Overhead Clap

Shoulder Taps with Reach Out

Shoulder Taps with Reach Up

Asymmetrical Arms

Alternate "V"Arms

Arm Punches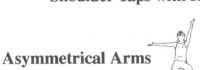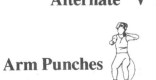

Front Foot Tap

Side Foot Tap

Leg March

Kick Out

Step Around Ball

Hop Around Ball

March-Arm and Leg

Unilateral Arms and Legs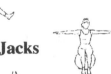

Cossack Dance

Half Jumping Jacks

Full Jumping Jacks

Sitting Skier

Arms and Legs In/Out

Open/Close Around Ball

Chapter 2

Side to Side Hip Roll

Front and Back Hip Roll

Circular Hip Roll

Gentle Trunk Rotation-Sitting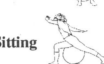

Advanced Trunk Rotation-Sitting

Supine Trunk Rotation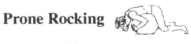

Prone Rocking

Kneel and Bow Stretch

Kneel, Bow and Side Bend

Side Stretch

Side Lying Trunk Rotation

Squat and Rock

Squat and Arch-Supported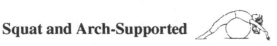

Chapter 3

Arm and Leg Lifts Quadruped

Gentle Upper Spine Extension Prone

Basic Push-Up

Airplane

Hip Lift-Spinal Mobility

Hip Lift with Bent Elbows-Spinal Mobility

Hip Lift with Raised Arms-Spinal Mobility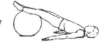

Hip Lift-Spinal Stability

Hip Lift with Bent Elbows-Spinal Stability

Hip Lift with Raised Arms-Spinal Stability

Advanced Hip Lift-Spinal Stability

Chapter 4

Gentle Abdominals-Sitting

Gentle Abdominals-Rotation

Abdominal Curls

Half Sit-Up Spinal Mobility

Half Sit-Up Spinal Stability

Half Sit-Up with Obliques Spinal Stability

Full Abdominal Curls

Dynamic Full Sit-Up

Dynamic Full Sit-Up with Obliques

Chapter 5

Ball Hug

Gentle Trunk Isometric-Supine

Push-Up

Advance Push-Up

Prone Walk Out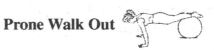

Total Body Flexion

Total Body Extension

Prone Skier

Log Roll

Hip Twister

Table Top Supine

Advanced Table Top Supine

Chapter 6

Hip Flexor Stretch

Hip Extensor Stretch Supine

Table Top Stretch

Hamstring Stretch Supine

Bent Knee & Hip Lift Spinal Mobility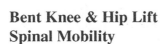

Bent Knee & Hip Lift Spinal Stability

Straight Leg Ball Lift

Frog Legs Supine

Leg Press-Supine

Leg Rotation with Ball

Side Lying Ball Lift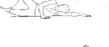

Side Stretch and Leg Lift

Push and Pull Sitting

Alphabet-Sitting

Alphabet-Standing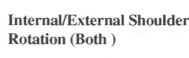

Chapter 7

Shoulder Flexion

Shoulder Extension

Shoulder Abduction

Active Assisted Horizontal Abduction

Active Shoulder Horizontal Abduction

Internal/External Shoulder Rotation (Single)

Internal/External Shoulder Rotation (Both)

Chapter 8

Ball Forward

Squat Ball Forward

Ball Overhead

Marching

Ball Sideways

Half Squat and Lift

Squat and Lift

Side Bend

Toss and Catch

Wall Squat-Body Mechanics

Glide-Extra Credit

Kneel Stand-Extra Credit

Chapter 9

Shoulder Horizontal Abduction

Shoulder Flexion to Elbow Abduction

Extension Forward

Shoulder and Elbow Extension

Elbow Flexion

Shoulder Flexion

Shoulder Abduction

Chop and Lift

Hip Abduction

Knee Flexion/Hip Extension

Prone Shoulder Flexion

Prone Shoulder Extension

Prone Shoulder Abduction

Chapter 10

Shoulder Blade Squeeze w/ Weights

Straight Arm Lifts-Side w/ Weights

Shoulder Extension w/ Weights

Alternate Arm Lifts w/ Weights

Elbow Extension w/ Weights

Shoulder Flexion w/ Weights

203

Glossary

Abdomen Belly, the part of the trunk that lies between the thorax and the pelvis.

Abduction Movement of a limb away from the central axis of the body

Adduction Movement of a limb toward the central axis of the body, or beyond it.

Active Assistive Patient assists therapist in range of motion when possible.

Asymmetry Lack of symmetry of parts on opposite sides of the body.

Balance Reactions Movement toward stability by automatically and appropriately adjusting the distribution of weight on each side of the vertical axis to maintain posture.

Base of Support Location on an object or body over which it's weight is distributed to maintain position.

Center of Gravity Point in the body that marks the force by which a body is attracted toward the earth by gravitational pull.

Cervical Relating to the neck in any sense.

Co-activation Activation of muscles surrounding a joint.

Connective Tissue The supporting or framework tissue of the animal body, formed of fibrous and ground substance with more or less numerous cells of various kinds.

Distraction Separation or "gapping" of joint surfaces.

Ergonomic A branch of ecology dealing with human factors in the design and operations of machines and the physical environment.

Extension Straightening a limb.

External Rotation Rotation away from the body's midline.

Flexion Bending a limb.

Hamstring Muscles The muscles in back of the thigh which bend the knee.

Inertia The state of a physical body in which it "resists" any force tending to move it from a position of rest or to change its uniform motion.

Internal Rotation Rotation toward the body's midline.

Isometric Static form of exercise when a muscle contracts without change in length or visible joint motion.

Kinematic Chain	Idea that all joints in the body are connected. Movement of one joint is accompanied by motion at an adjacent joint.
Lever Arm	The distance from a joint to the point at which a force is applied.
Lower Extremity	Leg
Lumbar	Relating to part of the back and sides between the ribs and the pelvis.
Mobilization	Making movable.
Momentum	The force of a moving object.
Oblique Muscles	Deep muscles of the abdomen whose fibers run diagonally from ribs to pelvis and cause trunk flexion and rotation besides stabilizing the spine anteriorly.
Percussion	A form of massage consisting of repeated blows or taps of varying force.
Perturbations	Something which causes a disturbance.
Prone	The body when lying face downward.
Proprioception	Information from sensory nerve endings concerning movements and positions of the body.
Quadriceps Muscle	Muscle in front of thigh which straightens the knee.
Quadruped	Position on hands and knees where the body weight is evenly distributed between the upper and lower extremities.
Reciprocal	To move alternately back and forth.
Rectus Abdominis	Superficial abdominal muscle which flexes the trunk and provides anterior stability to the spine.
Rotation	Turning or movement of a body around its axis.
Soft Tissue	Muscles and connective tissue.
Supine	Lying on the back.
Thorax	The chest; it is formed by the 12 thoracic vertebrae, the 12 pairs of ribs, the sternum, and the muscles and fasciae attached to these.
Upper Extremity	Arm
Vital Capacity	The volume of air the lungs can inspire.
Vertebra	One of the bones of the spinal column; there are usually 33 vertebrae, 7 cervical, 12 thoracic, 5 lumbar, 5 sacral (fused into one bone) and 4 coccygeal (fused into one bone).

Bibliography

Books

Amicarella, Marianna. <u>Dance Conditioning Handbook</u>. Louisville: Marianna Amicarella, 1994.

*Antoniotti, Terri and Mariano Rocabado. <u>Exercise and Total Well Being For Vertebral and Cranio-Mandibular Disorders</u>. IFORC. Tucson: Public International Fundamental, 1990.

Baviera, Dr. med Bruno. <u>On the Move</u>. Osoppo, Italy: Ledraplastic, 1994.

Baviera, Dr. med Bruno. <u>Rückenschmerzen-Anteitung Zür Selbsthilfe (Back Pain Instructions for Self-Help)</u>. CIBA-GEIGY, 1992.

*Bobath, Berta. <u>Adult Hemiplegia Evaluation & Treatment</u>. London: William Heinemann Medical Books Limited, 1978.

*Boehme, Regi, O.T.R. <u>Improving Upper Body Control</u>. Tucson: Therapy Skill Builders, 1988.

Butler, David. <u>Mobilisation of the Nervous System</u>. Melbourne: Churchill Livingstone, 1991.

Callaway, Paul, P.T. <u>Body Balance for Performance: Golf Exercise Program</u>. Elmhurst: Callaway Physical Therapy, 1994.

*Cooper, Douglas. <u>Dynamic Stabilization Exercises for the Lower Back</u>. Portland: Douglas Cooper, 1992.

Crabtree, Jeffrey and Diane. <u>Home Caregiver's Guide: Articles for Adult Daily Living</u>. Tucson: Therapy Skill Builders, 1993.

Cyriax, James. <u>Textbook of Orthopedic Medicine Volume One: Diagnosis of Soft Tissue Lesions</u>. Sixth Edition. London: Baillière Tindall, 1975.

*Davies, Patricia M. <u>Right in the Middle</u>. Heidelberg: Springer-Verlag, 1990.

*Dominguez, Richard H., M.D. and Gajada Robert. <u>Total Body Training</u>. New York: Warner Books, 1982.

Dvorák, Jirí and Dvorák, Václav. <u>Manuelle Medizin</u>. New York: Georg Thieme Verlag Stuttgart, 1985.

Fisher, Anne, Murray, Elizabeth and Bundy, Anita. Sensory Integration: Theory and Practice. Philadelphia: F.A. Davis Co., 1991.

Gray, Henry. Anatomy of the Human Body. 28th Edition. Goss, Charles Mayo (Ed.). Philadelphia: Lea & Febiger, 1966.

Headley, Barbara J. M.S., P.T., Cbt. The "Play-Ball" Exercise Program: A Stabilization Program for Back Pain & Dysfunction. St. Paul: Pain Resources, Ltd., 1990.

Hypes, B. Facilitating Development and Sensorimotor Function: Treatment with the Ball. Hugo: PDP Press, 1991.

*Keller, Lieselotte. Wirbelsäulen Gymnastik (Vertabral Column [Spine] Exercises). Falken: Falken-Verlag, 1992.

Kendall, Henry Otis, Kendall, Florence and Dr. Gladys Wadsworth. Muscles: Testing and Function. Baltimore: Williams and Wilkins, 1971.

*Kempf, Hans-Dieter and Dr. Jürgan Fisher. Rückenschule für Kinder (Back School for Children). Hamburg: Rowohlt Taschenbuch GmbH, 1993.

Kessler, Randolph and Hertling, Darlene. Management of Common Musculoskeletal Disorders: Physical Therapy Principles and Methods. Philadelphia: Harper and Row, 1983.

Klein-Vogelbach, Susanne. Ballgymnastik zur Funktionellen Bewegungslehre (Ball Exercises for Functional Kinetics). New York: Springer-Verlag, 1981.

Klein-Vogelbach, Susanne. Functional Kinetics: Observing, Analyzing and Teaching Human Movement. New York: Springer-Verlag, 1990.

Klein-Vogelbach, Susanne. Therapeutic Exercises. New York: Springer-Verlag, 1990.

Knott, Margaret and Voss, Dorothy. Proprioceptive Neuromuscular Facilitation: Patterns and Techniques. New York: Harper & Row, 1968.

*Kucera, Maria. Gruppengymnastik (Group Gymnastics). Stuttgart: Gustav Fischer Verlag, 1978.

Kucera, Maria. Gymnastik mit dem Hupfball (Exercises with the GymBall). 5th Edition. Stuttgart: Gustav Fischer Verlag, 1993.

Kucera, Maria. Krankengymnastische Übungen mit und ohne Gerät. Stuttgart: Gustav Fischer Verlag, 1988.

*Levy, Dr. Janine. The Baby Exercise Book. New York: Pantheon Books, 1975.

Lewit, Karel. Manipulative Therapy in Rehabilitation of the Locomotor System. 2nd Edition. Oxford: Butterworth Heinemann, 1991.

Maitland, G.D. Vertebral Manipulation. Fifth Edition. London: Butterworths, 1986.

Mayer, Tom and Gatchel, Robert. Functional Restoration for Spinal Disorders: The Sports Medicine Approach. Philadelphia: Lea & Febiger, 1988.

Moore, Dr. Josephine. Neuroanatomy Simplified. Cuernavaca, Mexico: Centro de Aprendizaje de Cuernavaca, A.C., 1988.

Orthopedic Physical Therapy, 2nd Edition. Donatelli, Robert and Wooden, Michael (Eds.). New York: Churchill Livingstone, 1994.

Porterfield, James and DeRosa, Carl. Mechanical Low Back Pain: Perspectives in Functional Anatomy. Philadelphia: W.B. Saunders Company, 1991.

Saunders, H. Duane. Evaluation, Treatment and Prevention of Musculoskeletal Disorders. Minneapolis: Educational Opportunities, 1985.

Schleichkorn, Jay. The Bobaths: A Biography of Berta and Karel Bobath. Tucson: Therapy Skill Builders, 1992.

Stedman's Medical Dictionary (23rd Edition). Baltimore: The Williams & Wilkins Company, 1976.

Sweet, Waldo E. Sport and Recreation in Ancient Greece: A Sourcebook with Translations. New York: Oxford University Press, 1987.

Webster's New World Dictionary (Third College Edition), Neufeldt, V. and Guralnik, D. (Eds.). New York: Webster's New World, 1988.

*Wilder, Brigitte. Sitzen Als Belastung ... wir sitzen zuviel (Sitting as Weight Bearing...We Sit Too Much). Zumikon: Verlag SVSS, 1991.

Periodicals

"Aktives Sitzen auf Gymnastikbällen zur Prävention von Haltungsschwächen im Primarschulalter" (Active Sitting on Gymnastic Balls for the Prevention of Posture Weaknesses in Primary School Age). Schweizer Physiotherapie Verband (Swiss Physiotherapie Journal). August 1991: 10-21.

Brody, Liz. "The Axler: A Workout That's Really on the Ball." SHAPE. April 1993: 86-93.

*Carriere, Beate, P.T. and Linda Felix, P.T. "In Consideration of Proportions." PT Magazine April 1993: 59.

Carriere, Beate, P.T. "Swiss Ball Exercises." PT Magazine September 1993: 92-100.

Day, Lee, P.T. "The Squat." Clinical Management November/December 1991: 81-82.

*Headley, B. "EMG and Low Back." Clinical Management May/June 1990: 18-22.

Irion, Jean M., P.T., A.T.C. "Use of the Gym Ball in Rehabilitation of Spinal Dysfunction." Univ. of Central Arkansas, 1992.

Lester, Merry, P.T. Spinal Stabilization and Compliance Utilizing the Therapeutic Ball: Case Study. Proc. of International Federation of Orthopaedic Manipulative Therapists. Vail, 1992. St. Augustine: I.F.O.M.T., 1992.

Marcks, Leslie Kent, P.T. "Clinical Suggestions: Using the Physio-Roll™ for the Facilitation of Motor Skills." Pediatic Physical Therapy. Fall 1993: 154-155.

*Morgan, D. "Concepts in Functional Training and Postural Stabilization for the Low Back Injured." Acute Care Trauma Rehabilitation. 2 (1988): 8-17

*Neuro-Developmental Treatment Association, Inc. Selected Proceedings from Barbro Salek Memorial Symposium, May 1984. Illinois: Neuro-Developmental Treatment Association, Inc., 1984.

Reichley, Melissa. "Roll With It: Swiss Ball Techniques." Advance for Physical Therapists. September 6, 1993: 10, 25.

Reichley, Melissa. "Aerobics Gets On The Ball" Advance for Physical Therapists. January 24, 1994: 5, 19, 20.

*Swaim, Kathleen, P.T. "An Alternative Therapy: Pilates Method." PT Magazine. October 1993: 55-58.

Urs, Illi. "Bälle statt Stühle im Schulzimmer?" Sporterzeihung in der Schule. June, 1994: 37-39.

Videos

Gomez, Ninoska, Ph.D. Refining Somatic Awareness and Mobility While Playing With Large Balls: Summary Report of an Experiential Research Project. Dèpartement D'èducation Physique, Universitè de Montrèal, November 1990.

Klein-Vogelbach, Susanne. <u>Functional Kinetics: Swiss Ball Exercises</u>. New York: Springer Verlag, 1981.

Lester, Merry, P.T. and Posner-Mayer, Joanne P.T. <u>Spinal Stabilization Using the Swiss Ball</u>. Denver: Ball Dynamics International, Inc., 1993.

Posner-Mayer, Joanne, P.T. <u>Orthopedic, Sports Medicine, & Fitness Exercises Using the (Swiss) Gymnic™ Ball</u>. Denver: Ball Dynamics International, Inc., 1991.

Posner-Mayer, Joanne, P.T. and Zappala, Lindsay. <u>FitBall™: The Balanced Workout</u>. Boulder: FitBall, U.S.A., 1993.

*Contains Swiss Ball information with other material.

Index

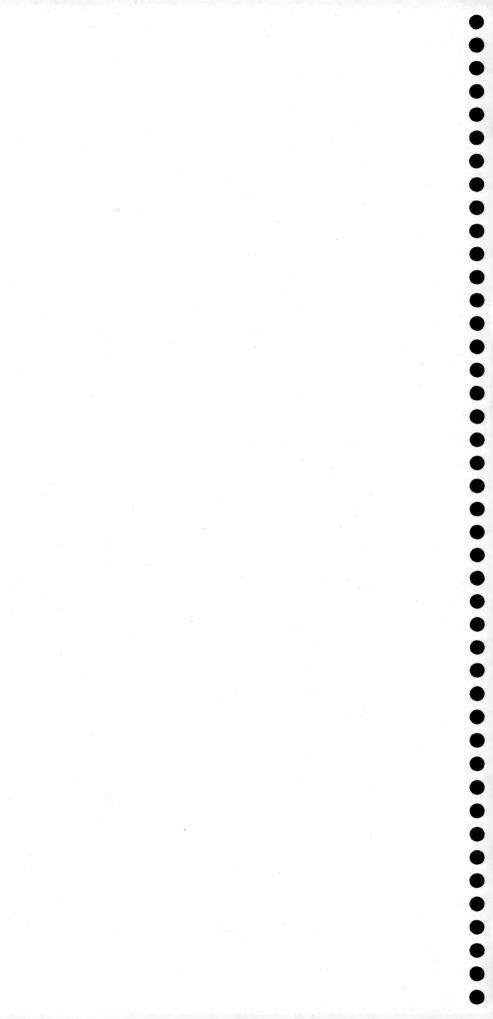